Advance Praise for Why We Forget
and How to Remember Better

"In *Why We Forget and How to Remember Better,* memory experts Andrew Budson and Elizabeth Kensinger provide readers with a practical and clearly explained masterclass on how memory works and how to keep it working well as we age. This is a must-read for anyone who wants to understand and maximize their memory functions."

—Wendy Suzuki, PhD, Professor of Neural Science and Psychology, New York University and internationally bestselling author of *Healthy Brain, Happy Life* and *Good Anxiety*

"In this highly readable book, two authorities on the science of memory and the brain unpack everything you could want to know about memory and memory disorders. You will find surprising answers here to fascinating puzzles—for example, why we form false memories, why someone with Alzheimer's disease remembers how to play the piano but forgets the names of family members, how to distinguish between memory decline due to normal aging and disorders of memory, and why sleep is so important for memory. In addition, the authors describe evidence-based ways to remember better and to defend against false memories."

—Ellen Winner, PhD, Professor Emerita at Boston College and author of the bestselling book *How Art Works: A Psychological Exploration*

"Budson and Kensinger have done a marvelous job creating an accessible summary of the wide-ranging field of memory research. A perfect place to start for anyone interested in understanding this fundamental human capacity."
—Joshua Foer, BA, Author of the bestselling book *Moonwalking with Einstein*

"This book delivers on all fronts. Written by two of the most eminent memory scientists in the world, the book draws in the reader immediately—engaging both the practitioners of the science of memory as well as those who are new to memory research. The reader is presented with many relatable, everyday examples and practical tips, and with concrete steps that unfold and explain complex theories of memory and forgetting. The authors cover a wide range of representative phenomena about when memory works and when it fails. The book delves into the neuroscience of memory and effects of aging at one end, strategies for improving memory at the other, and many key topics in between. I want this book for my memory course, and for my family and friends who are curious about how memory works."
—Suparna Rajaram, PhD, Distinguished Professor of Cognitive Science at Stony Brook University

"Everyone knows how memory works, we have our own experiences of remembering and forgetting to go on. But the science of memory, as Budson and Kensinger engagingly recount, teaches us so much more—how it really works and how it doesn't. And how this scientifically grounded knowledge enriches our understanding of our own minds."
—Ken Paller, PhD, Padilla Chair and Director of the Cognitive Neuroscience Program at Northwestern University

Why We Forget and How to Remember Better

The Science Behind Memory

ANDREW E. BUDSON, MD
Neurology Service, Section of Cognitive & Behavioral Neurology, & Center for
Translational Cognitive Neuroscience, Veterans Affairs Boston Healthcare System
Alzheimer's Disease Research Center & Department of Neurology
Boston University School of Medicine
Division of Cognitive & Behavioral Neurology
Department of Neurology
Brigham and Women's Hospital
Harvard Medical School
Boston, MA
Boston Center for Memory
Newton, MA

ELIZABETH A. KENSINGER, PhD
Department of Psychology and Neuroscience
Boston College
Chestnut Hill, MA

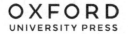

OXFORD
UNIVERSITY PRESS

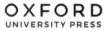

OXFORD
UNIVERSITY PRESS

Oxford University Press is a department of the University of Oxford. It furthers
the University's objective of excellence in research, scholarship, and education
by publishing worldwide. Oxford is a registered trade mark of Oxford University
Press in the UK and certain other countries.

Published in the United States of America by Oxford University Press
198 Madison Avenue, New York, NY 10016, United States of America.

Library of Congress Cataloging-in-Publication Data
Names: Budson, Andrew E., author. | Kensinger, Elizabeth A., author.
Title: Why we forget and how to remember better : the science behind memory /
Andrew E. Budson, M.D., Elizabeth A. Kensinger, Ph.D.
Description: New York, NY : Oxford University Press, [2023] |
Includes bibliographical references and index.
Identifiers: LCCN 2022027375 (print) | LCCN 2022027376 (ebook) |
ISBN 9780197607732 (hardback) | ISBN 9780197607756 (epub) |
ISBN 9780197607763 (ebook)
Subjects: LCSH: Memory—Popular works. | Memory—Physiological
aspects—Popular works. | Brain—Localization of functions—Popular works.
Classification: LCC QP406 .B83 2023 (print) | LCC QP406 (ebook) |
DDC 612.8/23312—dc23/eng/20220720
LC record available at https://lccn.loc.gov/2022027375
LC ebook record available at https://lccn.loc.gov/2022027376

DOI: 10.1093/oso/9780197607732.001.0001

This material is not intended to be, and should not be considered, a substitute for
medical or other professional advice. Treatment for the conditions described in this
material is highly dependent on the individual circumstances. And, while this material
is designed to offer accurate information with respect to the subject matter covered
and to be current as of the time it was written, research and knowledge about medical
and health issues is constantly evolving and dose schedules for medications are being
revised continually, with new side effects recognized and accounted for regularly.
Readers must therefore always check the product information and clinical procedures
with the most up-to-date published product information and data sheets provided by
the manufacturers and the most recent codes of conduct and safety regulation. The
publisher and the authors make no representations or warranties to readers, express
or implied, as to the accuracy or completeness of this material. Without limiting the
foregoing, the publisher and the authors make no representations or warranties as to the
accuracy or efficacy of the drug dosages mentioned in the material. The authors and the
publisher do not accept, and expressly disclaim, any responsibility for any liability, loss,
or risk that may be claimed or incurred as a consequence of the use and/or application
of any of the contents of this material.

Printed by Lakeside Book Company, United States of America

Contents

Foreword

In Christopher Nolan's gripping 2000 film *Memento*, protagonist Leonard Shelby seeks to find the man who he believes murdered his wife during a violent home invasion. Shelby's search is hampered by a head injury he suffered during the attack that resulted in a loss of his ability to remember ongoing events, making him dependent on handwritten notes, photographs, and even tattooed messages to himself in order to conduct the manhunt. Part of the film's genius is that Nolan presents the main plot by showing scenes in backwards order, so that the audience's experience is similar to Leonard's: Events unfold, but we have no idea what happened in the past that led to the present moment, requiring us to try to piece together the identity, role, and motives of the people we encounter.

Fortunately, watching *Memento* is about as close as most of us will ever come to experiencing life with a profound and unrelenting memory impairment. As someone who has spent his entire career studying memory, one of the reasons why I find *Memento* so compelling is that the film helps us to appreciate the enormous role that memory plays in our everyday lives, which we are liable to take for granted given how seamlessly our memory systems often work. Often—but not always. And that is why Andrew Budson and Elizabeth Kensinger's new book is so valuable. Memory can fail us in a variety of ways, with consequences ranging from mildly annoying to life-changing. If we can't recall the name of the actor who played Leonard even though we saw *Memento* and can picture the actor, we may be frustrated, but not much harm is done (the actor's name: Guy Pearce). Yet it is an entirely different matter if we forget to take an essential medication, can't recall information that is necessary to perform well on an exam, or incorrectly identify an innocent person as the perpetrator of a crime.

Psychologists and neuroscientists have built an impressive body of knowledge regarding the nature of remembering and forgetting, especially during the past few decades, and this scientific knowledge is essential for understanding how to combat the assortment of memory failures that can plague us. Budson and Kensinger are intimately familiar with this body of knowledge, and both of them have carried out research that has helped to expand our understanding of memory. Equally important, both have observed first-hand the everyday consequences of clinically significant forgetting. As a neurologist with expertise in Alzheimer's disease and other kinds of age-related memory impairments, Budson has seen up close what kinds of disruptions these impairments can cause in daily life. Kensinger is a psychologist who has worked with the most famous case of memory loss known to science—Henry Molaison, referred to in the research literature by the initials H.M. The forgetting that Henry experienced after surgical removal of brain regions that are now known to be essential for memory was so pervasive that he became the gold standard for memory impairment in the scientific literature, and likely a model for Leonard Shelby's character in *Memento*.

Building on their combined experiences, Budson and Kensinger are not only able to offer practical advice on how to combat various kinds of forgetting, but they also explain in easy-to-understand language why these lapses occur. By reading this book, you will come to see that some—perhaps many—of the ideas you had about memory are incomplete or flat-out wrong. You will see that memory is not a single thing, but instead composed of several distinct systems, each associated with a particular brain network. You will learn research-based strategies for making new memories and studying more effectively. You will gain insight into how emotion, exercise, sleep, and diet impact remembering and forgetting. You will become familiar with the differences between normal age-related forgetting and forgetting that results from Alzheimer's disease, and you'll understand why you should never tell anyone with Alzheimer's disease something that isn't true. You'll come to appreciate that forgetting isn't always a negative—we reap some significant benefits from forgetting.

You will also learn about one of the more fascinating aspects of memory, something that scientists have only come to fully appreciate in recent years, and an idea that my colleagues and I have worked on intensively: Memory isn't just about recalling the past; it also plays a crucial role in allowing us to imagine and plan for the future. This important function also underscores that memory is not simply a literal replay of past experiences; it is a far more dynamic constructive process that supports numerous cognitive functions. Memory's role in supporting these functions—ranging from planning to problem-solving to creative thinking—requires flexible processing; that is, the ability to use past experiences in new ways and in novel contexts. Memory is well suited to such tasks, but that same flexibility may also contribute to errors and distortions in remembering. As Budson and Kensinger discuss, these and other complexities of memory are intriguing and sometimes surprising, but researchers are studying them and are making progress in understanding their nature and basis.

Attempting to describe his strange mental condition to others, Leonard Shelby explained that although he could recall past experiences from before his head injury, he could not make new memories. "Everything fades," he mused. Alas, we are all susceptible to fading of memory over time, albeit to a much lesser degree than Leonard was. Understanding why it happens, and how to reduce or even stop forgetting when it interferes with our ability to perform everyday tasks, constitute important steps toward becoming a good steward of your own memory. Budson and Kensinger are just the right guides to take you on that journey.

Daniel L. Schacter, PhD
William R. Kenan Jr. Professor of Psychology,
Harvard University
Author of *The Seven Sins of Memory, Updated Edition: How the Mind Forgets and Remembers* (2021)
Newton, Massachusetts
January 2022

Preface

If you're like most people, you probably think you have a good, basic idea about how your memory works. After all, you use it daily to remember everything from your favorite childhood memory to last night's dinner—and all the "yesterdays" in between. You also use it to remember facts, like who Cleopatra and Harriet Tubman were, and what happened on July 4, 1776. And, of course, you use your memory when you practice piano scales and type on your phone with your thumbs without looking at the letters. So, if we asked you some basic questions about how memory works, your answers might include:

- My memory works like a video recorder; I record the information through my eyes and ears and then play the recording back in my head when I want to remember something.
- Memory evolved to remember information verbatim.
- When we forget things, it is a weakness of our memory system.
- When someone has amnesia, they typically cannot recall their name or identity.
- If someone can remember their childhood in vivid detail, they cannot be suffering from Alzheimer's disease.
- If one can play a musical instrument from memory without sheet music—and play it perfectly—they don't have dementia.
- When preparing for an exam, highlighting and re-reading important information is the best method of studying.

- Computerized brain-training games are an effective way to keep my memory strong for everyday activities.

Right? What if we told you that you're wrong? What if we told you that every one of those statements is completely wrong?

Don't worry if you were wrong; you're in good company. In 2011 the researchers Daniel Simons and Christopher Chabris found that most people they surveyed provided incorrect answers to questions like these.[1] It turns out that many aspects of our memories—and what happens to them when they break down—are simply not intuitive. Misunderstandings about memory can lead us to accept as true information that might really be false! That's one reason why distortions of memory—and outright false memories—occur so frequently even in perfectly healthy individuals.

WHY NOW?

Over the past 25 years, the fields of experimental psychology and cognitive neuroscience have revealed much about how memory works. We can now answer questions such as:

- Why did memory evolve? (Hint: It isn't simply to remember things.)
- How reliable is eyewitness testimony—and what influences its reliability?
- Why do false memories occur so commonly?
- How can a person with Alzheimer's disease remember how to play the piano but not their grandchildren's names (or even that they have any children)?
- What are the diets, physical exercises, and mental activities that have been scientifically proven to help keep your memory strong? (Hint: There are lifestyle changes anyone can make, and they don't need to cost a thing.)
- What are the most effective—and experimentally proven—ways to study for an exam?

- And how can you better remember daily information such as the name of the person you just met and where you parked your car?

FIVE PARTS

To provide you with the answers to these questions, we've divided this book into five parts.

In Part 1 we begin by explaining how memory is not actually a single ability but rather a collection of different conscious and nonconscious abilities. It turns out that remembering a phone number in your head, what you had for breakfast, the temperature at which water boils, and how to ride a bicycle use four different memory systems. We'll go through each of these systems, explaining how they work in your daily life. We'll finish with a discussion of collective memory, and what it means for a group of individuals—or even our whole society—to remember.

In Part 2 we focus on the heart of memory: how we remember the events that make up our lives. Here we dive into how we create, store, and retrieve memories of these events. We review the impact of emotion on memory. We discuss whether you can actually control what you remember and what you forget. And we discuss some of the interesting—and ordinary—circumstances in which memories can become distorted or just plain false. We also consider the relationship between confidence and memory, and how even if you are 100% certain of exactly where you were and what you were doing when you heard about the assassination of John F. Kennedy, the September 11th attacks, or the results of the 2016 presidential election, you may be mistaken.

Part 3 begins with how different neurologic and medical disorders like Alzheimer's disease, multiple sclerosis, epilepsy, Parkinson's disease, brain tumors, concussions/traumatic brain injuries, COVID-19, medical problems, anesthesia, hormone changes, and medication side effects can disrupt memory. We also review how psychiatric and psychological problems affect memory, such as anxiety, depression, attention-deficit/

hyperactivity disorder (ADHD), and post-traumatic stress disorder (PTSD). We end this part by discussing individuals who represent the other extreme—those with remarkable abilities to retain and recall information.

In Part 4 we review the changes to your lifestyle that can strengthen—or weaken—your memory, including the latest evidence regarding exercise, nutrition, alcohol, cannabis, drugs, sleep, social activities, music, mindfulness, as well as brain-training and other activities. We also talk about what doesn't work, including fad diets, phony medicines, and brain games that don't live up to their advertisements.

In Part 5 we discuss a variety of different memory aids and strategies to help you remember everything from your shopping list or French vocabulary to that presentation you need to memorize for work or the name of your colleague you haven't seen in 10 years. We'll explain how Mark Twain taught his children to remember the English monarchs and show you how to build your very own memory palace and remember 50 digits of pi.

We end the book by boiling it all down to some tips to help you remember better.

BUILT-IN SCIENCE FOR EVERYONE

To help you remember the main themes of this book, we've considered the science of learning when writing it. As we will discuss, repeating key ideas spaced out over time and interleaving different but related topics will facilitate your memory for information. For this reason, you might notice that some of the important topics are mentioned more than once. Rest assured that this minor repetition is intentional. We also use metaphors that can be concretely imagined—another strategy known to boost retention.

Spacing out your learning—and ideally sleeping in between learning sessions—can be helpful for optimal memory. So, if retaining the content in this book is a primary goal for you, we don't recommend that you read it all in one long sitting. Instead, try reading a few chapters, take some time to reflect on the content, and then return to it a little while later, perhaps after a night's sleep.

Because we've written this book for everyone, we used a variety of examples and metaphors to bring the text to life. We hope that whether you are at the beginning or end of your career, a student or an educator, or perhaps caring for your grandchildren or your grandparents, you'll find this book interesting, helpful, and memorable.

A WORD OF THANKS

Our first thanks go to Dr. Mary K. L. Baldwin, neuroanatomist, researcher, and artist, for creating the wonderful illustrations in the book. Our second thanks go to the many colleagues, students, friends, and family members who were kind enough to read and provide feedback and suggestions on the text, and to the student artists who aided us in seeing how our ideas could be visually represented; their insights helped to focus, clarify, and illustrate many key details and concepts. We also wish to thank our colleagues and the many individuals who trained in our research laboratories and clinics for conversations and exchanges that have inspired us to think in new ways about memory, to see new connections across studies, and to be excited about all that remains to be discovered.

Last but not least, we want to acknowledge our mentors in this field, Sue Corkin and Dan Schacter. Were it not for their pioneering research, much of memory would still be a mystery. And were it not for their patient mentoring of us, we would not be the memory teachers and researchers we are today.

Part 1

ALL THE WAYS TO REMEMBER

1

Memory is not one thing

One of us (Elizabeth) had the opportunity to conduct research with a gentleman named Henry Molaison (better known by his initials, H.M.[1]), who had the interior portion of his left and right temporal lobes (the part of your brain next to your temples) removed in 1953 because of epileptic seizures that were difficult to control. From a technical standpoint, the surgical procedures went fine. But, as he recovered, the doctors and researchers soon noticed something very troubling: He was unable to form any new memories. He could read, and talk, and if you were having a brief conversation with him, you would probably not notice anything amiss. But family members would visit and, although he knew who they were, he would have no memory of them coming. New doctors would introduce themselves and the next day (or even the next hour) he did not recall that he had met them. It was then that the doctors understood that, somehow, the removal of those parts of the temporal lobe caused him to become completely amnestic.

It was almost 50 years later when Elizabeth, then a graduate student, first met Henry in the laboratory of Suzanne Corkin at the Massachusetts Institute of Technology (MIT). By then, Henry had been to MIT many times, although he did not remember his prior visits. He would usually come

for a few days. On one day he might be asked to solve special crossword puzzles that would evaluate his memory for
words and concepts.[2] Another day he might complete some
tests of vocabulary and grammar rules.[3] On a third day he
might be asked to walk through a room several times and,
each time, remember a specific unmarked location on the
carpet.[4] Overnight, he would be cared for by the onsite
staff in the MIT university health services. Being amnestic,
someone would, of course, have to help him the next morning make his way from his sleeping quarters to Dr. Corkin's
laboratory.

During one of his visits, it was Elizabeth's job to guide Henry
to the laboratory. Left, right, right, straight, left, the corridors
continued through the maze of MIT's underground passage-
ways. Soon they came to a door, a door that was tricky to open,
and one that always gave Elizabeth a bit of trouble; you had to
hold one lever up while twisting the knob the correct direction . . . clockwise . . . or was it counter-clockwise? After observing her struggling with the door for a minute, Henry, always
wanting to be helpful, moved forward, performed the correct
complicated maneuvers on the door lock, and opened the door.

MEMORY SYSTEMS

How is it that an individual who is truly amnestic—someone
who, if you spoke with him for an hour, would not remember
meeting you 10 minutes later—can remember how to perform
the procedure to open a complicated door lock? There was
only one explanation for it, one that you may have deduced
yourself as quickly as the researchers who first worked with
Henry in 1953: Memory cannot be a single ability. Memory
must be a collection of abilities, only one of which is dependent upon the portion of the temporal lobes that was removed
in Henry.

It would not be an exaggeration to say that the contrast between Henry's profound amnesia for events and his normal ability to remember other things—such as knowing the set of motions needed to unlock the door—ushered in the modern era of memory research. We now understand that there are multiple memory systems in the brain, each with its own anatomical network that allows different types of information to be remembered. These memory systems can be classified in different ways, such as the timeframe in which they operate: short-term (seconds to minutes), long-term (minutes to several years), and remote memory (many years).

Long-term and remote memory systems are commonly further divided into those systems that are *explicit*, because conscious awareness is necessary for learning and retrieval, and those that are *implicit*, because conscious awareness (although sometimes present) is not needed for the learning and retrieval to take place. Explicit memory is often referred to as *declarative*, because it is easy to say or "declare" what you have learned, whereas implicit memory is also referred to as *nondeclarative*, because it is generally difficult to verbalize the memory.

A brief description of the principal memory systems follows; see also Figure 1.1. (Don't worry about the details; we'll have a separate chapter on each of the important systems.)

Long-Term and Remote Explicit/Declarative Memory Systems

- *Episodic memory* is memory for episodes of your life, such as how you celebrated your last birthday or what you had for dinner yesterday (Chapter 4). Episodic memory is often broken down into different parts such as creating, storing, and retrieving memories.
- *Semantic memory* is memory for facts and information, such as the color of a tiger's stripes, the purpose of a fork, and new vocabulary words in your Arabic language class (Chapter 5).

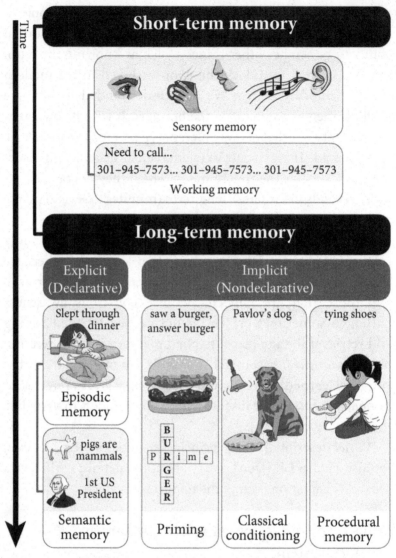

Figure 1.1. The memory systems that enable you to remember different types of information over different timescales.

Long-Term and Remote Implicit/Nondeclarative Memory Systems

- *Procedural memory,* sometimes called "muscle memory," is memory that you acquire by doing, including swinging a golf club, riding a bicycle, perfecting a yoga pose, and touch-typing on a keyboard (Chapter 2). Important components of procedural memory include the planning and coordination of movements.

- *Priming* occurs when a prior encounter with a particular item changes your response to the current item, whether you are consciously aware of it or not. For example, if you were doing a crossword puzzle and the clue was "American culinary specialty," you would be more likely to think of "hamburger" if you had recently seen an advertisement for McDonald's, whether you remember seeing the ad or not.
- *Classical conditioning* involves the pairing of two stimuli and was made famous by Pavlov's dog. When the unconditioned stimulus (the meat) is paired with the conditioned stimulus (the bell) a number of times, the response (salivation) may occur from the conditioned stimulus alone. This type of memory is important for traumatic and other highly emotional events, such as those that may lead to post-traumatic stress disorder (PTSD).

Short-Term Memory Systems

- *Working memory* allows you to actively keep information "in mind" and manipulate it, such as repeating a phone number silently to yourself while you find your phone to dial the number, following a mental route to avoid traffic, and calculating the tip in a restaurant (Chapter 3).
- *Sensory memory* refers to the momentary sights, sounds, smells, tastes, and tactile senses that impact your awareness, such as the color of a sunset, sound of a bird chirping, smell of coffee brewing, taste of a ripe peach, and feel of cool water on your skin (Chapter 3). Sensory memory quickly fades away—within 3 seconds or less—although some is transferred to working memory and some is eventually stored in episodic memory.

MEMORY SYSTEMS WORK TOGETHER

Having stated clearly that our memory abilities rely on a collection of distinct memory systems that process different information for different purposes, we must state equally clearly that, in daily life, multiple memory systems typically act together, simultaneously storing information and events in multiple ways and brain regions. It is also true that none of these memory systems are completely independent; they all interact with and—in many cases—depend upon each other.

For example, when you listen to a new song, the sensory memory in your ears and sound processing parts of your brain become active, storing the sounds of the song for a few seconds—long enough that the sounds can be transferred to your working memory system. As you are using your working memory and consciously thinking about the song (perhaps noting the amazing guitar solo), your episodic memory will automatically kick in and lay down a memory for where you were (in your car) and what you were doing (heading to dinner with friends) when you heard this song. Your episodic memory will also link the melody of the song with its name.

The next morning as you're dressing, you hear the song again. Your episodic memory immediately recalls not only the name of the song but also where and when you heard it: driving to have dinner with friends. You download the song and listen to it on your way to work. As you continue to hear the song in various places and times over the next month (in the grocery store, waiting in line for coffee, walking in the park) a new semantic memory is forming, linking the melody of the song with its name, such that when you hear the melody it brings to mind its name, and not one of the 20 or so individual times that you heard it.

By the end of the month, you decide you're going to learn the song on your guitar. You find the sheet music online, read the first couple of bars, and keep the notes "in your head" using your working memory. F, E, D, E, B, D, G, F, you repeat silently to yourself as you play the notes on your guitar, teaching your fingers which frets to press and strings to strum as your procedural memory learns the motor movements required to play the song.

One day you get a minor cut on your finger. For a few days, every time you play a particular chord, the string rubs against the cut, and you experience a brief moment of pain. The next week, the cut has healed, yet you find your body still preparing for that brief jolt of pain every time you place your fingers in position for that chord. Classical conditioning has occurred, creating the association between that chord and the pain in your finger. Only after a couple of pain-free practice sessions does that association begin to fade.

MEMORY SYSTEMS DEPEND UPON EACH OTHER

These examples illustrate the interdependence of the memory systems. Sensory memory is a necessary precursor of just about all memory, as most of what you remember comes in through your senses. Although episodic memory is essentially "always on," such that you don't need to try to remember the events of your life (it just happens), any time that you are intentionally trying to remember information (such as where you parked your car or the quadratic equation), you need to use your working memory to focus your attention on the information. If you want to acquire some new facts (such as the name of a new restaurant or the conjugation of a Spanish verb), you need to first remember them using your episodic memory; only later (and generally through multiple episodic memory events) do the new facts become part of your semantic memory.

Some of the most interesting memory phenomena occur when there is a divergence in what our different memory systems remember, such as when we "forget" an event from our episodic memory but still "remember" the event using a different memory system. For example, at one point Andrew was feeling quite pleased with his guitar playing, having learned a new song in record time with minimal difficulty. It was only when he proudly mentioned this achievement to his guitar teacher that he was reminded that they had already worked on that song 3 years earlier! So, although his procedural memory system remembered the song—allowing him to relearn it quickly—his episodic memory system had forgotten that he previously learned it.

It can also happen that you forget the episodic memory associated with a prior emotional trauma, but its effects remain through classical conditioning. Let's suppose that as a teenager you discover that—despite having no difficulties with roller coasters, Ferris wheels, drop towers, and haunted houses—you are absolutely terrified of merry-go-rounds. In fact, you can't even approach a merry-go-round without breaking into a cold sweat. It's only when you mention this strange phenomenon to your mother that she tells you the story of how when you were 4 years old, a circus clown tried to comfort you on a merry-go-round ride but ended up scaring you half to death. She then further explains that this is why they never took you to amusement parks during the rest of your childhood.

* * *

Now that you understand how your ability to remember stems from a collection of memory systems—partly separate but also partly dependent upon and interacting with each other—we're ready to examine each system individually. We will begin with procedural memory, the memory system that allowed Henry Molaison to unlock that complicated door for Elizabeth.

HOW TO HELP YOUR MEMORY SYSTEMS WORK TOGETHER

You can use the different memory systems in your brain together when learning and retrieving information. Using multiple memory systems will create strong and long-lasting memories.

- When you want to use episodic memory to remember the details of an event you are experiencing, pay attention to information coming through your senses into sensory memory.
  - To form a strong episodic memory of a birthday celebration, focus on the sights of the cake, candles, presents, and the people at the party. Enjoy the sounds of the singing and the laughter. Savor the taste of the chocolate cake. Notice how the champagne bubbles tickle your nose.
- When you want to learn new semantic memory information, try manipulating the information in working memory. This manipulation will help to form a strong episodic memory that will, in turn, help you to form a long-lasting semantic memory.
  - To learn new vocabulary words, use your working memory to actively think about different aspects of the word and its meaning. Consider the syllables and the unusual spelling of onomatopoeia. Think about how it describes words like "sizzle," "crackle," and "squish." Imagine yourself listening to the "boom" of a cannon, the "meow" of a cat, and the "tick-tock" of an old clock.
- To acquire a new skill, use your episodic memory to learn the instructions that will eventually be internalized in your procedural memory.
  - To learn to touch-type using procedural memory, you need to first use your episodic memory to memorize where you should place your fingers on the keyboard, which keys each finger should reach to, and that your thumb will press the space bar. Only then are you ready to practice, enabling your procedural memory to learn the correct fingering, which brings us to Chapter 2.

2

Procedural memory

Muscle memory

Today's the big day: You're going to teach your 6-year-old daughter how to tie her shoes. She's ready for you, standing there with her shoes on, the laces falling loosely to the floor. She looks up at you expectantly.

"First, you cross the laces," you say as she does it. "Then, you . . ."

You pause because you suddenly realize you're not sure what the next step is!

You look down at your own shoes, untie the knot, and retie it slowly, observing—and memorizing—each step in the sequence as you do it. Only then do you continue, "OK, now take the top lace, loop it under and around the bottom lace, and pull it through."

MUSCLE MEMORY = PROCEDURAL MEMORY = SKILL LEARNING

How is it possible that, after tying your own shoes almost every day since you were her age, you couldn't explain to your daughter how to do it? Why did you need to untie your own shoes and study how you retied them to be ready to teach her the

next steps? The simple but surprising answer is that you were
lacking some aspects of memory for how to tie your shoes—you
did not have an explicit (conscious), declarative (you can say it
aloud) memory. OK, you argue back to us, maybe it's true that
you couldn't explain aloud how to tie your shoes but, of course,
you *know* how to tie your shoes—you do it every day. And this
apparent paradox brings us to the topic of this chapter.

Procedural memory is an implicit (unconscious), nondeclarative (difficult to verbalize) memory system used for procedures,
routines, sequences, and habits that you acquire by doing. It is
also referred to as *skill learning* (because it is the memory system you use to acquire and improve skills) and sometimes as
muscle memory (because it often appears as if the muscles are
doing the learning). We will see, however, that this latter term
is a misnomer; it is most definitely regions of the brain—not the
muscles—that are remembering the skills we learn, such as riding a bicycle and playing a musical instrument. In fact, we use
procedural memory when we engage in some predominantly
mental activities such as adding a column of numbers and writing out a check.

ACQUIRING NEW SKILLS

You have developed many skills and habits without the intent
to learn—such as turning a door knob and opening the door, or
knocking twice on wood for luck. Other procedures you have
learned intentionally—such as using chopsticks or driving. For
these latter procedures and skills, the learning often occurs in
three stages.

In *stage 1*, the instructions are said aloud (or written out)
to the extent possible. If you are learning to drive, you may
hear the instructor say, "First adjust the seat so your right
foot can comfortably reach both pedals. Familiarize yourself with the foot pedals; the left one is the brake, the right

one is the accelerator. Use only your right foot to press the pedals. Adjust your side- and rear-view mirrors so you can see to either side of the car and behind you through the rear window. Put your seatbelt on. Start the car ignition with the key or button. While keeping your right foot on the brake, release the emergency brake. Still keeping your right foot on the brake, move the gearshift lever from Park to Drive (or Reverse). Slowly take your foot off the brake and feel the car start to move . . ."

Stage 2 occurs after you've learned the correct sequence of the basic actions, whether through reading instructions, watching others (or videos), or listening to the teacher sitting next to you and giving you instructions. In stage 2, you need to concentrate and think of the actions—using your episodic memory to recall the steps and your working memory to go over them in your mind—while you are performing the skill. So, as a new driver, every time you get into the car, you're thinking to yourself, "Adjust the seat. Adjust the mirrors. Seatbelt on. Right foot on brake. Start the car ignition. Move the gearshift lever. Slowly take my foot off the brake . . ."

By *stage 3*, you're doing all the actions in the correct sequence automatically, without thinking about them. Your episodic and working memory are no longer needed. Instead, your mind is free to think about other things, such as what you need to get at the grocery store or the conversation you're having with your friend sitting in the passenger seat. It is only when conditions are unusual—such as an icy road—that you need to consciously think about your driving.

Wait a minute, you say: How do you get from stage 2 to stage 3? How do you go from needing to say the steps in your mind to it occurring automatically? The answer can be summed up in one word: *practice*. Practice is what allows you to go from stage 2 to stage 3, and more practice allows you to gain expertise at your new skill.

Practice, Practice, Practice

There's an old joke that goes like this: A musician carrying a violin case stops a New York City taxi driver and asks, "How do you get to Carnegie Hall?" The driver leans out the window and says, "Practice, practice, practice." And, of course, the taxi driver is correct: The best way to improve your skills, whether on the piano keys, the basketball court, or the yoga mat, is to practice. Practice is the key to improving your skill, and extensive practice is required to achieve expertise.[1]

FEEDBACK

Well, that seems simple enough: To improve a skill, you need to practice it. But what's the best way to practice? For starters, you need to make sure that you are practicing the skill correctly and moving toward your goal—otherwise you'll learn the wrong thing. So, you'll need some type of feedback to know when you're doing it right and when you're not. Now if you are practicing throwing darts, the feedback may be immediate: You can see how far the dart lands from the center of the target. This feedback may be all you need to improve your throws. Perhaps after practicing 7 hours in your first week, you can hit the target 10% of the time. At the end of the month, you've improved to being able to hit it 25% of the time. Another month, and you're up to 30%. Three months later, you're at 33%. Six months after that, you're still at 33%. Hmm . . . you seem to have reached a plateau, where additional practice isn't giving you more improvement. This is a common phenomenon you've probably experienced. For most skills, you can improve only so far on your own. That's where coaching comes in.

COACHES AND TEACHERS

Coaches can provide feedback not only on how far you are from hitting the target, but also on your *technique* in achieving your goal. A coach can instruct you to watch the ball as it's coming to you, to hold the dart lightly in your hand, to look at the whole chessboard before you make a move, and to keep your numbers lined up straight in the columns when you're learning long division. Videos and other instructional materials can also be helpful if you have not mastered the basics, but once you have, there is no substitute for a teacher who can look and see what you are doing right and what you are doing wrong as you strive for your goal.

SPACE IT OUT AND SLEEP ON IT

OK, so you now know that to improve on a skill you should practice it and use feedback and coaches to help you reach your goal. What's that you're saying? You already knew all this? Hold on, we're just getting to some of the most interesting—and nonintuitive—parts of procedural memory.

Let's say you want to improve your free throws. You have your basketball and access to a 10-foot-high hoop with a regulation backboard. You're willing to put in 7 hours each week to practice. The feedback is immediate—the ball either goes through the hoop or it doesn't—and you've got a coach who is helping you to improve your technique each week. So, how should you divide up the 7 hours each week? Should you practice for an hour a day? Or should you really focus on your throws and do it all on Saturday, 3.5 hours in the morning and afternoon, with a lunch break in the middle?

If you tried both options, the studies suggest that you would feel more satisfied with your performance after the all-day-Saturday option versus the an-hour-a-day option. But in this case your intuition would be wrong. The studies clearly show that you will benefit more from the same hours of practice if you space it out, practice 1 hour each day, and sleep between sessions.[2]

CAN YOU KEEP LEARNING BETWEEN PRACTICE SESSIONS?

There are a number of interesting factors that may explain the benefit of spacing out your practice sessions rather than doing all your practicing at once. One of them is that your skills may actually be improving between practice sessions—that's right, your skills may be improving even when you're not practicing or thinking about the skill. This "offline" learning can occur both during the day while you are awake and overnight while you are sleeping, although the offline learning may be more robust and less susceptible to interference while you are sleeping.[3]

Another way that you can continue to improve between practice sessions is to review the skill you are learning in your mind. This may involve mental imagery if you picture yourself jumping up, releasing the ball, and watching it swish through the hoop. Or you may imagine other senses as you feel the violin against your chin and the strings on your fingers as you pull the bow across with your other hand and hear note after note burst forth. Studies have shown that individuals who engage in mental imagery can improve their motor skills in everything from ping pong to delicate surgical procedures.

WATCH OUT FOR INTERFERENCE

Now that you know that skill learning may be improved between practice sessions with offline learning, it may not surprise you to hear that you may inadvertently disrupt this offline learning by performing a similar yet different practice session the same day. For example, let's say that although you have never played a racquet sport in your life, you won a free 1-month membership at a racquet sport club that includes tennis, squash, and racquetball. Wanting to make the most of your free membership, you sign up for three lessons each day—tennis in the morning, squash at noon, and racquetball in the afternoon. Is this a good way to learn? Well, although you're spacing the learning out for the three sports and sleeping between lessons, your noon squash lesson is going to interfere with some of what you learned on the tennis court that morning, and your afternoon racquetball session will interfere with both your tennis and squash lessons. So, it might be best to just concentrate on one sport for that month and really master it, enabling your offline learning to improve your skills without interference.

START SLOW AND PRACTICE DIFFERENTLY

Winter is here and you're absolutely determined to master that double black diamond ski slope that you had so much trouble with last year. So, this year, you've decided that you're going to ski down that slope not 5, not 10, but 15 times every time you go out skiing. That will give you the best chance of mastering it, right?

It turns out that in most circumstances varying your practice is better than practicing the same way every time. Because the snow conditions, prior skiers, lighting, temperature, humidity, wind, and other factors are going to be different every time you ski down a slope, no two ski runs will be the same. On any given day the snow may be fine and powdery, thick like oatmeal, full of glare ice, or loose and granular. If you want to be able to ski down that double black diamond slope with confidence in any condition, you can actively seek out areas of the mountain with all of these different types of snow and practice on them.

Moreover, one of the best ways to vary your practice is to start slow and gradually increase the difficulty. This means that to give yourself the best chance of mastering the double black diamond slope, you want to warm up on the easiest green slopes, practice on the intermediate blue slopes and really master *them*, then do some of the expert single black diamond slopes, and finally practice that double black diamond slope.

Similarly, when learning new pieces, most musicians begin by warming up on scales, then practice the new music at a slower pace than it would normally be played, before increasing the tempo to the appropriate speed. Not only does gradual training generally lead to better overall performance, but also less total effort is required than if you tried to achieve the same level of mastery by practicing on the most difficult task every time.

DO YOU NEED TO PRACTICE IF YOU'VE GOT TALENT?

Some people appear to have a talent or gift that enables them to learn a skill more quickly. But practice is essential to bringing out everyone's full potential, regardless of talent. With greater practice, individuals with seemingly little innate talent can progress farther than so-called prodigies. There is also evidence that practice can bring out individuals' genetic potential. The more they practice, the more similar the performance of identical twins becomes, while the performance of fraternal twins diverges.[4] The bottom line is that whether you believe you are the next Mozart or just the second violin, the only way to find out just how good you can become is to practice.

DO PROCEDURAL MEMORIES LAST A LIFETIME?

There's a saying that once you've learned to ride a bike you never forget. But is that actually true? Yes and no. Yes, procedural memories, including skills like riding a bike, can last a very long time—often much longer than most episodic and semantic memories for events and facts, respectively. Nonetheless, skills do deteriorate over time if you don't practice them. So, don't expect to be able to play that guitar solo as well today as you did 30 years ago if you haven't touched your guitar between then and now. In fact, although the rate of loss of procedural memories is less than we see in episodic and semantic memories, the pattern of decay is similar, such that the decay is rapid at first, then slows down, and finally becomes fairly stable. In other words, when you're not playing your guitar, your soloing ability drops considerably in the first weeks and months, becomes a bit worse over the next year or two, and then declines more slowly after that. The good news is that whenever you do decide you'd like to go back to the guitar, it won't take you that long to get back to where you were before.

THE BASE NODE, THE LITTLE BRAIN, AND THE BRAIN'S BARK

If you wish to avoid irksome anatomical terms with Latin names, feel free to skip over this section; we promise you'll still understand what comes next. But we find it fascinating that skill learning has its own anatomical system. Its separate anatomy is one reason scientists consider procedural memory to be its own memory system. There are three brain regions that are particularly important for skill learning: the *basal ganglia* (Latin for *base node*), the *cerebellum* (Latin for *little brain*), and the *cerebral cortex* (Latin for *brain's bark*, its outer covering); see Figure 2.1.

Although it is widely accepted that these three brain structures are essential for the acquisition and use of skills, it turns out that this little system is wildly complex. We don't yet understand precisely how the system works together, or exactly what the roles are of the basal ganglia versus the cerebellum. We'll give you a small taste of some of the findings that are known, even if there isn't enough information to draw a clear picture (metaphorically and literally).

Your basal ganglia, deep in the center of your brain, may be particularly important for stimulus–response interactions (such as seeing a red STOP sign and automatically pushing the brake pedal). For example, individuals with damage to the

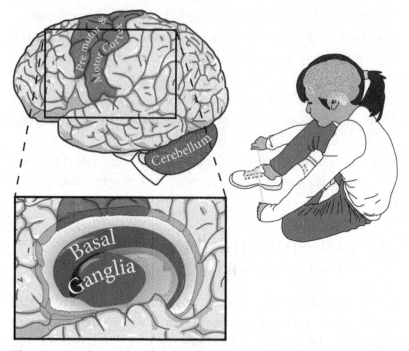

Figure 2.1. Procedural memory involves the cerebellum and basal ganglia as well as the premotor and motor cortex. Box in lower left shows a cutaway view of the basal ganglia deep inside the brain.

basal ganglia were slower to learn both motor and non-motor reaction-time tests.[5] Similarly, cells in the basal ganglia change their firing pattern when a skill or pattern is learned—even if the learning is purely mental and has no action involved with it, such learning your multiplication tables.[6]

Your cerebellum, in the back of your head just above your neck, may be particularly important in skill learning that involves precise sequences and timing, including acrobatics, dancing, and tracking a target. Proper function of the cerebellum is considered critical for a high level of performance in competitive sports. The cerebellum is also critical for many cognitive and emotional functions,[7] and thus it is also involved in the learning and use of non-motor skills as well.

Your cortex, the outer covering of your brain, is involved in most cognitive and motor functions that require a high level of precision for control or discrimination. Cortical regions involved with finger and hand movement have been found to be expanded and reorganized in violinists and racquetball players.[8] In fact, changes in the cortex can be observed as soon as 1 week after training on a task. And if the training involves sensation instead of motor skills (reading Braille, for example), it is the sensory cortex that becomes reorganized.

BRAIN DISEASES CAN DISRUPT PROCEDURAL MEMORY

Not surprisingly, the brain diseases that impair procedural memory are those diseases that can disrupt the basal ganglia, the cerebellum, the cerebral cortex, or their connections with each other and other brain regions. Such disorders include Parkinson's disease, dementia with Lewy bodies, strokes, tumors, and multiple sclerosis, among others. See Chapters 13 and 14 for more information.

You may be interested to know that patients with more typical, episodic memory disorders—including Henry Molaison (H.M.), who was discussed in Chapter 1, and those with mild Alzheimer's disease—can usually learn procedural memory tasks without difficulty. Why is this the case? Because impairment of episodic memory is caused by damage to different brain regions, as we will discuss in Chapter 4.

IS MINDFULNESS A PROCEDURAL MEMORY SKILL?

These days, many people routinely engage in one or another type of meditation, including mindfulness, where you practice observing the mind, particularly as it wanders (as it tends to do), even as you gently bring it back and attempt to focus your attention in the present moment. As with other activities, if you work at being mindful, of course you'd like to get better at it. Which brings up an interesting question: Is mindfulness a skill that can be practiced and improved upon like any other procedural skill? We think the answer is probably yes. We've saved this section for last because it is a bit more speculative than everything else discussed in this chapter.

Why would mindfulness be considered a skill? Certainly, people talk about mindfulness skills, training, and practice, and if you've practiced mindfulness at one time or another, you can easily recognize that training your mind takes work like any other type of training, and you might notice yourself moving through the stages of skill learning.

So, why wouldn't mindfulness be considered a skill? Mostly because it doesn't really have an objective and outwardly observable outcome that you can measure, such as how many free throws you can get through the hoop in a row, how fast you can ski down that slope, or even how many digits you can add up in your head.

One way to help determine whether mindfulness is a skill is to look at the brain regions that are active when one is learning mindfulness. Are the brain regions activated with mindfulness training those that are known to be activated with skill learning and procedural memory? Or those that are known to be activated with other types of learning such as episodic and semantic memory?

The convergent answer from many studies is that mindfulness training activates a variety of brain regions and networks, including those active in procedural memory, such as the basal ganglia and cerebellum.[9] That the procedural memory network is not the only one involved is a good reminder that memory systems almost never act in isolation, but with both other memory systems and other brain functions such as attention, sensory processing, emotion, reasoning, and judgment.

HOW TO IMPROVE PROCEDURAL MEMORY SKILLS

Now that you understand how procedural memory works, improving your skills that use procedural memory is fairly straightforward:

- Work on learning the right way the first time so that you don't have bad habits that you need to correct.
  - So, rather than trying to learn how to play the guitar or tennis on your own, take lessons.
- Once you know the right thing to do, practice, practice, practice. As long as you are practicing correctly, all skills improve with practice.
- Use feedback to improve your practice and your performance.
  - Whether from a teacher listening to your clarinet playing or a stopwatch timing your 100-meter dash, feedback is essential to ensure that any changes you are making in your practice are bringing you closer to your goal.
- Whatever skill you are doing, continue working with a teacher or coach for optimal performance.
- Space out your practice to optimize offline learning.
  - If you're practicing a total of 7 hours each week, it's much better to switch to doing 1 hour each day rather than 7 hours in 1 day.
- Minimize interference by avoiding practicing another similar skill the same day that may interfere with what you wish to learn.
  - In other words, if you're determined to learn the Lindy Hop, don't try to learn another dance later in the day.
- When you practice, start with an easier task and build up to the more difficult ones.
  - Do some basic skating and single jumps before you tackle your double axel/triple toe loop combination.
- Vary your practice so that you will be able to perform at your best under a variety of conditions.
  - To improve your chances of the ball going through the hoop, practice your three-point shot from different places around the line.
- Lastly, it's so important we'll say it a few more times: Practice, practice, practice.

3

Working memory

Keep it in mind

Your friends have nominated you to place the group's order at the juice and smoothie bar. "I'll get the Zany Zucchini," one of them shouts out. "I'll have Java Journey," another says. You silently repeat the orders in your head, "One Zany Zucchini and one Java Journey." Your friends continue saying orders and you add them to the list you're silently repeating over and over. You enter the long line as you continue saying to yourself, "Zany Zucchini, Java Journey, Purely Pineapple, Wheatgrass Wonder, Best Banana, Matcha Mango, Chunky Chocolate."

Finally, it's about to be your turn, when someone cuts in line and starts to place their order. You are so astonished and outraged that it takes you a minute to realize that the server behind the counter has told them to go to the back of the line and is now waiting for you to place your order. You step and say, "Thanks. I'll have one Zany Zucchini, one Java Journey, and, and . . ." And you can't recall the other five drinks.

Has this ever happened to you, a time when you were able to keep track of a bunch of items in your head by silently repeating them—only to lose them when you were interrupted? If so, you've experienced some of the power and the fragility of *working memory.*

MAINTAINING AND MANIPULATING CONSCIOUS INFORMATION

Working memory is the ability to maintain—and manipulate— information that you are consciously thinking about. Not only does working memory allow you to keep lists of drinks, phone numbers, and directions in your head after someone tells you the information, but it also allows you to manipulate and use that information to achieve your goals.

For example, to decide which of two sweaters you should buy, you need to both keep key bits of information in mind that are relevant, and you also need to compare the features in order to make the best decision. Your working memory can keep in mind the features of one (100% wool, looks puffy, will keep you warm) and the other (mixed materials, latest style, may need to wear a jacket with it) and help you to compare them.

This ability to temporarily store and manipulate information for your own goals and purposes is quite powerful; in other words, you can put working memory to work for you! Unlike long-term memory, however, the information in working memory must be consciously attended to. If attention is interrupted—as in our list of drinks example—the information will be lost.

Now that you understand the basics of what working memory is and how it can be useful, let's look at some of its details, keeping the following questions in mind: How does information get into working memory? How much information can you store? How do you keep it there? How do you manipulate it? How does information flow from working memory into long-term memory and vice versa? What brain structures are involved in these processes? Which diseases disrupt working memory? And lastly, what can you do to improve your working memory?

MOVING INFORMATION IN

Sensory Memory

As we mentioned briefly in Chapter 1, *sensory memory* is memory of your sensations—the momentary sights, sounds, smells, tastes, and tactile senses that impact your awareness. Let's consider an example.

As you start to take a bite of the apple, you first experience the smooth, slightly waxy feel of your lips pressed against the skin, and then the sensation of the pressure required by your teeth to pierce it. Then, as your teeth break through, the juice bursts into your mouth and the sweet, tart, and slightly spicy taste of the apple flashes into your consciousness. You're then aware of the texture of the flesh of the apple on your tongue, perhaps mixed with that of the peel. You chew for a minute and swallow, experiencing a feeling of contentment as the apple makes its way into your stomach.

For a split second you can actually remember each of these sensations perfectly, in addition to the apple's shiny red color with some patches of green at the top as you spied it in your friend's fruit bowl, its firmness in your hand as you picked it up, and the satisfying crunch you heard as you bit into it. These sensory memories fade within seconds, however, unless you decide to think about these sensory experiences. If you do think about them, you've transferred them into working memory.

Retrieval from Long-Term Memory

Now that you have these sensations in your working memory, any one of them may provide a cue that triggers the retrieval of one or more long-term memories into your consciousness— that is, into your working memory. For example, along with the sensations of the apple you just bit into, you can also bring up memories of other apples that you have eaten into your working memory so you can compare their tastes with this one. You first consider the McIntosh, but its skin and flesh are softer than your apple. Perhaps the Red Delicious? No, it's sweeter than yours. Maybe the Golden Delicious? The texture is similar, but the color is all wrong. Finally, you recall the color, taste, and texture of the Macoun, and realize it is a perfect match with the apple you're eating.

So, another way to bring material into your working memory is to retrieve information from your long-term memory. In fact, every time you retrieve and consciously think about a memory for a fact (your granddaughter's birthday is April 15) or an event (her second birthday party last week), you are bringing it into your working memory. Once it is in your working memory, you can examine its various aspects (she was so light when you picked her up) and use that information for a purpose (she's probably a size 2T; that's the size outfit you'll purchase for her) or just to enjoy and reexperience the emotion of the event (her smile melting your heart).

THE MAGICAL NUMBERS 7 AND 4

Do you know why phone numbers are seven digits (without the area code)? It's not by accident. It comes from research that was made famous by Harvard psychologist George Miller in 1956 in his article "The Magical Number Seven, Plus or Minus Two."[1] Miller observed that most young adults could keep about seven digits in their working memory, although some could store only five, and others as many as nine.

Several decades later, Nelson Cowan at the University of Missouri and other researchers showed that the reason seven digits can be kept in working memory is because most of us automatically "chunk" numbers into sets of two digits, and we can keep three or four chunks of information in mind.[2] But you can train yourself to remember even more information. If you happen to know that 212 is an area code of New York City, you can keep that in mind as a single piece or chunk of information. In fact, a pair of researchers were able to train an individual to keep 80 digits in his working memory by chunking them into numbers that he was familiar with—race times because he was a runner.[3] We'll talk more about chunking in Chapter 8.

THE PHONOLOGICAL LOOP AND VISUOSPATIAL SKETCHPAD

In 1974, two research psychologists from England's University of York, Alan Baddeley and Graham Hitch, proposed a model that included separate systems for keeping verbal and visual information in working memory. Verbal information, they suggested, is maintained by silently repeating the information to yourself in what they termed the *phonological loop*. (Think of the juice drinks example at the beginning of this chapter.) Visual information, by contrast, is maintained by the *visuospatial sketchpad*. (Examples include following a route in your mind or visualizing where the knob is on your front door.) With only minor modifications, this model with its separate systems is currently used today.[4]

One reason the phonological loop and visuospatial sketchpad are considered separate storage capacities for working memory is that each can keep track of about three or four chunks of information. So, it's possible to think about chunks of verbal information and also chunks of nonverbal images in your mind at the same time. Note, however, that if you start silently labeling the images to yourself (this abstract painting looks like a cityscape and that one looks like giraffes), then you'll be impinging upon your verbal working memory capacity.

WHERE ARE WORKING MEMORIES ACTUALLY STORED?

Left Versus Right Hemisphere

Another reason that this model incorporating separate systems for verbal and visual working memory is useful is that it maps onto where the memories are actually being stored in the brain. As you may know, your left brain is specialized for verbal information and your right brain for images and other nonverbal information. So, when you are using your phonological loop and silently repeating your grocery list in your head, that is occurring primarily in your brain's left hemisphere. When you are going over a map in your mind of the best route to get to your aunt's house, that is occurring primarily in your brain's right hemisphere.

What about if you're left-handed? Do these lateralization rules still apply? It turns out that this dominance is reversed in only 7% of left-handed individuals (right-brain dominant for verbal information, left-brain dominant for visual information), although in 22% of left-handers and 12% of right-handers there is no strong dominance (verbal and visual information roughly equal in both hemispheres).[5]

While these lateralization differences hold true in most people, the last thing to say about left versus right hemispheres is that both hemispheres actually contribute to verbal and visual working memory most of the time. For example, when you talk silently to yourself, the words themselves are coming from your left hemisphere and the tone of your silent voice is coming from your right hemisphere. And when you look at a map in your mind, although your right hemisphere is paying attention to all of it, your left hemisphere is also paying attention to the right side of the map and is rehearsing the names of landmarks or streets.

Where in the Hemispheres?

OK, so we know that verbal working memory storage is taking place primarily in the left hemisphere and visual working memory primarily in the right hemisphere. But each hemisphere is a fairly large place—almost half your brain. The question naturally arises: Where in the hemispheres is the information in working memory being maintained?

Each hemisphere comprises four lobes, and it turns out that the same lobes that are active when you're perceiving or doing something are also active when you are imagining perceiving or doing it in your mind. So, if you are silently repeating a list of juice drink orders to yourself, it is the same language areas in your left hemisphere that are active as if you were saying the information aloud. More specifically, it is a special part of your frontal lobe that performs speech (called Broca's area) that is silently saying the words, and it is the part of your brain that performs hearing further back and just above your ears in your temporal lobe that "hears" the silent words. Similarly, if you are following a map to your aunt's house in your mind, it is the same areas in the very back of the brain in the occipital lobes that are active as if you were actually looking at the map.

OTHER MODALITIES OF WORKING MEMORY

Now that you understand a bit more about keeping verbal and visual information in mind using your phonological loop and visuospatial sketchpad, you might be wondering about other modalities of working memory. After all, doesn't the composer keep musical notes, phrases, and melodies in mind? Doesn't the perfumer imagine and recombine a variety of scents? Doesn't the gourmet chef mentally consider how a new combination of ingredients prepared in specific ways would taste together? We speculate that these other modalities of working memory occur as well, and that they are stored in the same place in the brain where the perceptions of these sounds, smells, and tastes are processed. In fact, we can even think of a "movement working memory" when an athlete reviews the actions they perform when they swing a bat or perform the breaststroke, and mentally makes some modification to their swing or stroke.

CHOOSING, EVALUATING, AND MANIPULATING INFORMATION: THE CENTRAL EXECUTIVE

Having explained how you get information into working memory and maintain it there, we will now turn to how you can manipulate information in working memory to enable your reasoning, judgment, problem-solving, and planning.

Just like a business needs a CEO—a chief executive officer—to make the important decisions and lead the company to successfully achieve its goals, your working memory needs a central executive. The central executive chooses what information to bring into working memory, how to evaluate it, when to manipulate it, and finally what movement or other activity it should direct the rest of the brain (and body) to do (see Figure 3.1).

Top Down Versus Bottom Up

Your central executive works for you—it helps you achieve your goals. If your goal is to win a game of chess, your central executive helps you focus your attention on the board, diminishes your awareness of other things in the environment, and enables you to plan your next move. Your central executive can actually move the chess pieces around in your mind, allowing you to try out alternative moves by using and manipulating the information of the chessboard on your visuospatial sketchpad. Note that this focusing of attention can work so well that neither the insect buzzing nearby nor the people speaking at the next table even enter your consciousness.

There are times, however, when you want to be interrupted—even in the middle of your chess game. There may be external

Central Executive   Visuospatial Sketchpad

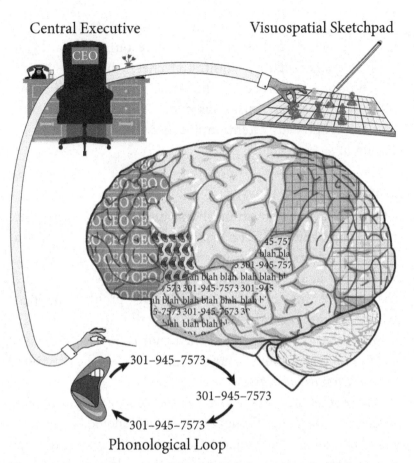

Phonological Loop

Figure 3.1. In the model proposed by Alan Baddeley and Graham Hitch, the prefrontal cortex serves as the central executive ("CEO" pattern) of working memory that coordinates both the visuospatial sketchpad (grid pattern) in the parietal and occipital lobes and the phonological loop (open mouths and "blah 301-945-7573" pattern) in the frontal and temporal lobes.

stimuli that are important to pay attention to, such as the smell of smoke and sight of flames erupting from the kitchen. Or perhaps it is a more subtle but still important internal signal, one that tells you that you must excuse yourself in the next 3 minutes and head to the washroom or you're going to have an embarrassing accident.

Thus, in a *top-down* manner, your central executive directs attention and other processing resources toward your explicit goals (such as winning at chess), but also decides which *bottom-up* processes that arise from visual, auditory, olfactory, or other sensations should reach consciousness and interrupt your attention because you may need to act on them.

Don't Be an Old Horse

There's a saying that an old horse always follows the same route. Have you ever been driving while engrossed in a conversation (or perhaps your own thoughts) and ended up where you usually drive to, such as school or work, rather than where you intended to go? This problem happens because your central executive was allocating your conscious attention (sometimes called your *controlled processes*) to your conversation or your thoughts and left the driving to your *automatic processes*.

So, another important task for the central executive is to determine when your thoughts and actions should be on "autopilot" and when you should be consciously thinking through one or more steps as you are doing them. In fact, large portions of our actions each day do occur automatically without much conscious thought. One common example is your morning routine. Getting up, using the toilet, brushing your teeth, showering, toweling off, brushing your hair, dressing, getting into your car, and even driving to work are all processes that occur relatively automatically with little conscious input. You may consciously pause to consider which shirt or outfit to put on depending upon what meetings you have on your calendar that day, but then you go back on autopilot as you slip your arms through the sleeves, button up your shirt or blouse, and tie your shoes.

Other Activities of the Central Executive

Your central executive is also actively involved in almost every purposeful, deliberate, conscious activity that you undertake. Here are a few more examples:

- Doing arithmetic in your head.
- Inhibiting your automatic response to pet a friendly-appearing dog that you don't know.
- Focusing your attention to find a friend you are meeting in a crowded park.
- Being able to switch back and forth and have simultaneous conversations with your spouse and your toddler, both of whom are clamoring for your attention.
- Keeping track of the errands you need to do.
- Planning the most efficient route to travel to get your errands done.
- Developing strategies to help you accomplish your goals—and changing your strategies if they are no longer working.
- Determining the individual steps that you will need to accomplish to achieve your larger goals.

As you can see, your central executive enables you to do a variety of complicated activities that require conscious thought. These activities include short- and long-term planning as well as other goal-oriented behaviors.

MULTITASKING

No one is able to do two activities at the same time as well as they can if they just focus on one of them—period, no exceptions. Having stated this clearly, you may have noticed that there are some things you often can do simultaneously (reasonably well) and other things that you simply cannot do at the same time. With the information you have learned in this chapter thus far, you are now ready to understand why that is the case and which types of activities you are likely to be able to do together—and which you are not.

Keep in mind the following three points that we have reviewed:

1. Some processes can occur automatically without your constantly devoting conscious attention to them. These automatic processes generally operate using *procedural memory* (often referred to as habits, routines, or skills), as we discussed in Chapter 2.
2. The central executive of your working memory system is needed to consciously interrupt and override these automatic processes any time you need to do something different from your usual routine.
3. You have two main working memory storage systems, your phonological loop for verbal information and your visuospatial sketchpad for visual information.

What Happens When You Multitask

Let's say that you're driving toward your workplace but you're not going there—it's Sunday and you're going to a park to meet a friend for a walk. To reach this park, you need to turn off the main road earlier than you would to reach your workplace. You're looking at the road you're driving on and you are consciously thinking about that right turn you need to make in about 10 miles. Let's consider three different scenarios.

- *Scenario 1*: You're watching the road and the landmarks as the miles go by, saying silently to yourself, "I need to remember to make that right turn." You slow down appropriately and make the turn, reaching the park a few minutes later.
- *Scenario 2*: You're driving on the road, and your mobile phone rings. Keeping your eyes on the road, you answer it with a button on the steering wheel. It's your daughter, and she is excitedly telling you about a surprise award she won earlier that day. As she describes the award and the events leading up to it, you pull into

the parking lot at your workplace—only then realizing that you missed your turn toward the park.

• *Scenario 3*: You're driving on the road, and your mobile phone rings. After your daughter briefly tells you about a surprise award she won, she asks for Grandpa's number so she can call him as well. Keeping your eyes on the road, you work to remember the number. You are thinking of your little paper phonebook that you keep in the kitchen. You can see the page in your mind. His number is in the bottom right-hand corner. It begins 978 . . . CRASH! You hit the car in front of you. (Luckily, no one was hurt.)

OK, so let's consider what happened in each scenario. In *Scenario 1*, you used your verbal working memory (your phonological loop) to help you pay attention, and so your central executive was able to turn off the "autopilot," alter your usual driving routine, and make the correct turn to reach the park. In *Scenario 2*, your verbal working memory—and hence your conscious attention—was diverted to your conversation with your daughter. You can't both repeat something silently to yourself and have a conversation with someone. In addition, your central executive was now thinking about what to say in the conversation rather than the route you were traveling. For both of these reasons, you stayed on autopilot, missed the turn, and ended up at your workplace. In *Scenario 3*, both your verbal and visual working memory were diverted to your conversation, forcing your central executive to work particularly hard as it tried to toggle between the information stored in the verbal and visual codes. Moreover, your automatic visual processes were impaired because you cannot both use your working memory to recall a visual image and see clearly what is in front of you at the same time. Your brain's visual system—busy focusing on retrieving the image from your kitchen phonebook and putting it into your visuospatial sketchpad—was unable to correctly perceive the car in front of you (interpret its speed, judge its position, etc.), and so you didn't slow down in time.

Multitasking Take-Home Messages

First, anytime you are trying to concentrate on two things at once, your attention for each will be diminished relative to your focusing your attention on just one thing at a time. Second, although your performance on each will be diminished, you may still be able to do two things at once if one of them is automatic and the other, conscious one is in a different modality (verbal vs. visual) such that it uses a different part of the brain. Third, you will always experience great difficulty if you try to perform two tasks that both use the same brain system—that is, you'll always be impaired if you try to do two verbal or two visual tasks at the same time.

INTERACTIONS BETWEEN WORKING MEMORY AND OTHER MEMORY SYSTEMS

Working memory rarely acts alone. At the beginning of this chapter, we explained that when you retrieve an *episodic memory*, a memory for one of the events that make up your life (such as your granddaughter's second birthday party), you are bringing that episodic memory into your conscious, working memory. Similarly, when you were trying to determine what type of apple you were eating, your central executive was bringing up the knowledge stored in your *semantic memory* of one variety after another (McIntosh, Red Delicious, Golden Delicious) until you hit upon the correct one (Macoun). We also discussed how another important job of your central executive is to decide when to let those activities run by your *procedural memory* (such as dressing or driving) proceed automatically, and when to consciously interrupt and direct them (wear best suit for job interview today; remember to drive to the park and not to work).

The Gateway to Long-Term Memory

Your working memory is also the gateway to long-term episodic and semantic memory. Most of the information that eventually makes its way into your episodic and semantic memory stores is initially kept in mind and consciously considered by your working memory. This is probably most obvious if you think about studying something—such as vocabulary words in your Arabic language class. It is your conscious, effortful engagement with the material in working memory that leads to its ultimate storage in semantic memory.

For episodic memory, as we'll discuss more in Part 2, although you can remember an event without that being your goal, you do have to consciously attend to it in working memory in order for it to enter your store of event memories. Have you ever been riding in a car and not been able to recall anything about the scenery for the last 5 minutes despite the fact that your eyes were open and pointed out the window? The usual reason is that you were using your working memory to daydream about something else. Because you consciously attended to your daydream in working memory, your daydream itself can enter episodic memory—in fact, you might be able to remember that specific daydream for the rest of your life. But you'll never be able to recall the scenery you passed because it didn't enter your working memory.

Google Your Long-Term Memory

Your working memory—and specifically your central executive—can also help you to search for knowledge in your long-term episodic and semantic memories. For example, if you're trying to recall the last restaurant you ate at, your central executive could use the strategy of querying each of your meals, starting with the most recent one and working backwards, to find the one you ate at a restaurant. Or, your central executive could think about all of your favorite restaurants and determine which of those you ate at most recently. Or, perhaps it might use a geographic strategy, and think about those restaurants closest to your home, expanding outward until the one you ate at most recently is identified.

So, in brief, the central executive is responsible for transferring information back and forth between working and long-term memory, linking several of our different memory systems together. Does it seem silly that we're speaking of the central executive in the third person? It is "you," of course, but the point we're trying to make is that now you know which part of you is actually doing this work—your central executive. Which brings us to our next question: Just where in the brain is this clever central executive?

THE PREFRONTAL CORTEX

There is a growing consensus that the central executive and its remarkable abilities, including planning, foresight, decision-making, judgement, and related behaviors, are located in the prefrontal cortex—that is, in the frontmost part of the frontal lobe. It is well connected to the rest of the brain, enabling its "command and control" functions. The prefrontal cortex takes up about 33% of the human brain, while making up only 4% of that of the cat, perhaps explaining why humans appear to have a wider repertoire of goal-directed activities than their feline companions. Moreover, there is also a gradient in the frontal lobes themselves regarding how abstract or "big picture" the activities are, with the more abstract ones in the front and the more concrete ones in the back.[6]

As an example, let's say you want to watch the sun rise where its rays first touch the United States on the summer solstice. This very abstract goal would be in the frontmost part of your prefrontal cortex. To accomplish this goal, you need to climb to the top of the 1,748-foot mountain named Mars Hill in New Brunswick, Maine, near the Canadian border. This less abstract goal would be a bit further back in your prefrontal cortex. To accomplish the goal of climbing the mountain, you need to continue hiking up the trail in front of you, which would be toward the back of your prefrontal cortex, as it is a fairly specific, concrete goal. Note that these are not three different steps or stages of your journey—these are three different ways to conceptualize what your goals are at that moment. Another example that naturally comes to mind as we are writing these words is that we have the fairly abstract goal of writing this book, which includes the progressively more concrete goals of writing this chapter, this section of the chapter, this paragraph, and this sentence. (Writing specific words, typing specific letters, and moving our fingers to push down on the keyboard also take place in the frontal lobes but are so concrete that they are further back, behind the prefrontal cortex.)

One way that this abstract-to-concrete gradient is relevant is in the instructions that you need to give children of different ages whose frontal lobes become progressively mature and connected to the rest of their brain as they age.[6,7] For example, you can ask a 14-year-old to "Make a sandwich," and, if they like peanut butter and jelly, they will get out the bread, peanut butter, jelly, plate, knife, and (hopefully) a napkin and make themselves the sandwich. For a 6-year-old you will probably need to say, "Take out the bread, peanut butter, and jelly. Now take out a plate, knife, and napkin. Put two pieces of bread on the plate. Spread peanut butter on one side of one piece, jelly on the other side of the other piece, and put them together."

WHAT DECREASES WORKING MEMORY?

Brain Disorders That Disrupt Working Memory

Now that you understand that the prefrontal cortex—the front part of your frontal lobe just behind your forehead—is where the central executive of working memory is located, it should not surprise you to learn that any brain disorder that disrupts the frontal lobes or its connections to the rest of the brain will disrupt working memory.

Brain disorders that may damage one or more regions of the frontal lobe include strokes, tumors, multiple sclerosis, and head trauma. There are also a number of neurologic disorders that affect the frontal lobes more diffusely, including cerebral palsy and dementia (such as behavioral variant frontotemporal dementia, vascular dementia, and normal pressure hydrocephalus). Most individuals who have one of these brain disorders affecting the frontal lobes either show diminished working memory capacity or impaired ability to evaluate and manipulate information. Psychiatric disorders can also affect working memory, including depression, attention-deficit/hyperactivity disorder (better known by its initials, ADHD), and psychotic disorders, such as schizophrenia. We will briefly discuss all of these disorders in Chapters 13 and 14.

Anxiety and Stress

Anxiety and stress interfere with working memory for at least two reasons. The first is that when you're anxious or stressed, you may find yourself thinking about and preoccupied with whatever you are anxious or stressed about. If your phonological loop is busy repeating statements like, "I'm never going to be able to get through this presentation," your ability to use your verbal working memory to remember your presentation will be impaired. And if you're silently repeating, "Everyone is staring at me because of my bad haircut," you'll have difficulty paying attention to what people are actually saying to you. Similarly, if your visuospatial sketchpad is full of frightening images of a big, red "F" on your final exam, you'll have difficulty picturing your notes where you outlined the correct answer.

The second reason that stress interferes with working memory is due to the changes that occur in your body. There are hormones released into your bloodstream, such as adrenaline, that trigger your "fight or flight" response. This response forces you to pay attention to those things in your environment that could represent a threat, even if those things have absolutely nothing to do with what you are trying to accomplish at that moment. Thus, your working memory capacity may be taken up by your fear of forgetting the lines of your soliloquy—which actually prevents you from remembering the lines.

WAYS TO IMPROVE YOUR WORKING MEMORY

After having reviewed working memory and how it functions, now you're ready to improve your ability to direct your central executive to pay attention, keep information in mind, and manipulate that information to achieve your goals.

- Pay attention.
  - Attention is the foundation of working memory, so there is nothing more important than paying attention if you are trying to improve your working memory.
- Don't multitask!
  - Turn off your cellphone, the television, and other distractions when you are trying to keep information in mind.
- Focus on your sensations.
  - Start by focusing on your sensations and keeping them in mind if you want to remember the sights, sounds, tastes, smells, and touches that you are experiencing.
- Chunk information together when needed to keep it all in mind—particularly if there are more than three or four parts.
  - Whether the information is verbal or visual, you'll be able to keep more of it in mind if you chunk pieces of it together, such as fruits, vegetables, and meats on a shopping list. For more on chunking, see Chapter 8.
- Relax and don't be anxious.
  - You're going to have difficulty keeping information in mind if you are anxious or stressed. If you have a tendency to be anxious, consider using mindfulness meditation or deep breathing to help you feel calmer and more relaxed. That way you will be

able to focus on what you want to—rather than what you are anxious about.

- Drink a cup of coffee (or tea).
  - ○ Although you don't want to be anxious, neither do you want to be too laid back. You want to be alert, attentive, and not sleepy when you are trying to keep information in mind. Sometimes a cup of coffee or tea can help you to be more alert and pay attention better.
- Improve your active attention by practicing mindfulness.
  - ○ Practicing mindfulness meditation is one way to improve your ability to consciously, actively, pay attention to what you want to. See Chapter 21 for more information.

4

Episodic memory

Travel back in time

A 75-year-old man came to the clinic with his daughter because of memory difficulties. Although he believed that his memory problems were due to normal aging, his daughter was more concerned. Despite being a wonderful grandfather who typically kept track of his grandchildren and what they all were doing, he didn't remember the birth of a new grandson last month. She also noted that for the past 2 to 3 years he has been getting lost while driving and would tell the same stories to the same people again and again. In fact, it seemed that his old high school stories were the only things he wanted to talk about. His memory for those remote events appeared to be excellent—which confused his daughter. After relating this history, her first question to us was, "How can his memory be so good for things that happened 60 years ago when he can't remember what happened yesterday or last month?"

RIBOT'S LAW

How indeed? This astute question by this patient's daughter was also posed more than 100 years ago by the French psychologist Théodule-Armand Ribot. As discussed in his 1882 book *The*

Diseases of Memory, Ribot realized that memory loss generally follows a pattern that has become known as Ribot's law.[1]

Starting from the onset of the brain injury—whether from trauma, dementia, or other causes—Ribot observed that individuals will show:

- Impaired ability to form new memories
- Impaired ability to recall recent memories
- Preserved ability to recall remote memories

Explaining Ribot's law will be just one of the interesting aspects of *episodic memory* that we will discuss in this chapter.

YOUR PERSONAL TIME MACHINE

You can think of episodic memory as your own personal time machine. Episodic memory allows you to travel back in time in your mind to a prior event or *episode* of your life, such as your first kiss or where you had dinner last evening. When you use your episodic memory, you can often see the scene in front of you, feel the emotions that made your pulse quicken, and experience your other senses vividly as if you were there again, looking out through your eyes. It is, in fact, this subjective experience of being present in the memory that helps us to define episodic memory. But before we are ready to understand how we can retrieve a memory and travel back in time, we need to first understand a bit about how episodic memories are built in the first place.

ENCODING EPISODIC MEMORIES

Encoding is the word we often use to describe when an event enters into our memory. The word correctly implies that the event is being turned into a *code*. Your sensory stores might initially register the information, but in order to remember the sights you are seeing, sounds you are hearing, tastes you are savoring, thoughts you are thinking, and emotions you are feeling for an event in your life, you must then pay attention to these details using your *working memory* as described in Chapter 3. Each of these sensations, thoughts, and emotions occurs in particular brain regions. For example, vision mainly occurs in the occipital lobes in the back of the brain. Thinking in words involves a loop including part of your frontal lobe that silently says the words and the upper part of your temporal lobe that "hears" the silent words. Once in working memory, the neural pattern of activity that makes up that experience can travel from these parts of the brain that do the sensing, thinking, and feeling to a special structure on the inner aspect of your temporal lobe.

THE SEAHORSE IN YOUR HEAD

Put your fingers on your temples, the sides of your head just behind your eyes. Now slide your fingers back until you reach your ears. If you drew a line between your fingers, you would pass through the inner part of your temporal lobes that contains the *hippocampus*. Hippocampus is Latin for seahorse, and this structure is named for it because it has a head, slender body, and curved tail that together look a little bit like a seahorse (if you spent too much time in the anatomy lab). As we will discuss next, the hippocampus is where episodic memories are formed.

STORING THE MEMORY

Several important things happen to the neural code for the pattern of activity that represents the sights, sounds, tastes, thoughts, emotions, and other experiences that make up an event of your life when it enters your hippocampus. The first outcome is that these separate sensations, thoughts, and

emotions become bound together in a coherent representation. This binding allows the memory for the entire event to
be stored and later retrieved. The second outcome is that this
bound representation becomes tagged with an index that will
allow you to retrieve and reactivate the memory at a later time.

For example, let's consider your memory for breakfast one
morning. You slip on your fuzzy slippers, get the coffee brewing,
and start to make yourself an omelet with eggs, cheddar, pep-
pers, and onions. Despite the exhaust fan, the kitchen is soon
filled with the smell of the onions in the frying pan. As you sit
down in the morning light, sip your coffee, and have your first
bite of the omelet, you glance at the newspaper headlines and
learn that one of your favorite musicians has died. You turn on
the radio and, not surprisingly, they're playing *Imagine*, one of
his songs. You listen with a sadness in your heart. The neural
activity related to the disparate sensations, thoughts, and emotions related to this episode of your life—from the sight of the
headlines in your occipital lobes to the sound of the song in the
upper part of your temporal lobes—is transferred to your hippocampus, where it becomes bound together and indexed for
later retrieval.

RETRIEVING THE MEMORY

A week later you're sautéing some onions as the first step in
your chili recipe. Your kitchen becomes filled with the aroma of
onions frying. The neural activity related to this aroma travels
from the nerve endings in your nose, through the part of your
brain that processes smell, and into the hippocampus. The pattern of activity related to this particular odor of frying onions
happens to be a near-perfect match with that of your breakfast last week. This pattern match acts as a cue that triggers the
retrieval of your prior episodic memory. Not just the smells
but the entire bound representation of the memory with all
of its sensations, thoughts, and emotions is retrieved, actively

recreating the sights, sounds, tastes, and feelings you experienced during the original memory episode of making breakfast the prior week. In fact, the same parts of your brain that processed your sensations when you were originally experiencing the event are now working to replay those remembered sensations. Soon the upper part of your temporal lobes are "hearing" the song *Imagine* and your occipital lobes are "seeing" the newspaper headline announcing that John Lennon is dead.

INDEXING THE MEMORY

Now that you understand the basics of storing and retrieving episodic memories, let's dive in a bit deeper to better understand just how the binding and indexing of memories occurs. Imagine you are going to park your car in the same parking garage on three successive days. How is it that are you able to find your car each day? And why is it often difficult to do so?

This particular parking garage has two floors (first and second) and two sections (red and blue). We're also going to use how you are feeling each day to indicate your mood as well as other important contextual details that may differ from one day to the next.

- *On the first day*, you park your car on the first floor, in the red area, and you smile as you pull into a spot halfway down the aisle on the left, as there was little traffic. This event's set of circumstances (first floor, red section, feeling happy) leads to a distinct pattern of brain activity that allows you to create a unique hippocampal index that, in turn, allows you to easily find your car at the end of the day.
- *On the second day*, you park your car on the second floor, in the blue area, and you frown as you pull into a spot halfway down the aisle on the right, as the traffic has made you late for your meeting. Nonetheless, this distinct set of circumstances (second floor, blue section, feeling upset) leads to a distinct pattern of brain activity that again allows you to create a unique hippocampal index that will enable you to easily find your car.

- *On the third day*, you also park your car on the second floor, in the blue area, and again you frown as you look at the time and pull into a spot all the way down the aisle on the left. This event's set of circumstances is quite similar to that of yesterday (second floor, blue section, feeling upset). We would like to have a new hippocampal index form that will help us to remember that we parked our car on the second floor, in the blue area, and all the way down the aisle on the left, but we have a problem.

When there are highly overlapping circumstances leading to highly overlapping patterns of brain activity—as there are for the second and third days—a separate hippocampal index will not form. Instead, you'll have a single hippocampal index for days two and three. This single index will be strengthened for what the two memories have in common, but will be unclear for the aspects that differed. So on the third day it will be easy for you to recall that you parked your car on the second floor in the blue area, but it will be difficult for you to remember whether you parked it halfway down the aisle on the right, or all the way down the aisle on the left.

BEYOND THE SEAHORSE

At this point you have a good, basic understanding of how the hippocampus allows us to store and retrieve memories. There are, however, other brain regions that contribute to episodic memory in important ways. As we will see, the frontal and parietal lobes are also needed for episodic memory function.

The Prefrontal Cortex in Episodic Memory

Do you recall the *central executive* located in your prefrontal cortex (just behind your forehead) from Chapter 3? We described it as the CEO of your working memory system. As information needs to first get into working memory before it can get into episodic memory, it shouldn't surprise you that the prefrontal cortex and its central executive are also critical for the proper functioning of your episodic memory system. We'll be discussing episodic memory in great detail in Part 2, so here we'll simply list some of the key actions of the prefrontal cortex in episodic memory to illustrate its important role:

- Chooses the goals of what information you wish to remember.
- Directs attention so that information can enter working memory and then episodic memory.
- Aids in remembering the context for the information.
- Helps to remember the order in which information was learned.
- Chooses the goals of what information you wish to retrieve.
- Directs the search to retrieve information from your episodic memory.
- Develops strategies to help you retrieve information.
- Helps you evaluate the accuracy and applicability of the information you have retrieved.

Similar to working memory, the left prefrontal cortex and left hippocampus are more involved in storing and retrieving verbal information, and the right prefrontal cortex and right hippocampus are more involved with storing and retrieving visual and other nonverbal information (see Figure 4.1).

Conscious Recollection: The "Aha!" Moment

Have you ever been searching your memory for information and, when it finally appears, you think to yourself, "Yes! That's the information I've been looking for"? It turns out that this conscious, vivid experience of recollection occurs in the top back part of your brain called the *parietal lobe*.[2] Perhaps for this reason, investigations into memory using magnetic resonance imaging (MRI) scans almost always show parietal lobe activation when memories are retrieved.

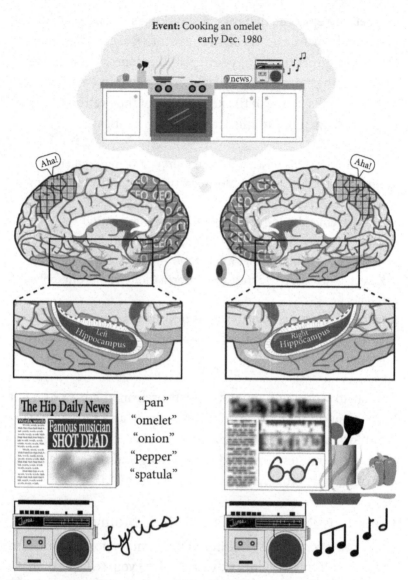

Figure 4.1. Memory for a single event arises from the two hemispheres working together: the left hemisphere for verbal information and the right hemisphere for images and other nonverbal information. Eyes indicate front of the brain, near the frontal lobes ("CEO" pattern). The parietal lobe creates the "aha" moment when you consciously retrieve a memory (grid pattern). Boxes show cutaway views of hippocampus deep inside the temporal lobe.

DISORDERS OF EPISODIC MEMORY

If we consider the roles played by the hippocampus, frontal lobes, and parietal lobes in episodic memory, it should be possible to understand the effects of many brain disorders. Individuals whose hippocampus is damaged or removed, such as Henry described in Chapter 1, will experience difficulty forming new memories and retrieving recent memories but (following Ribot's law as discussed at the start of this chapter) will still be able to retrieve remote memories. Those who have damage to frontal lobes or its connections—from traumatic brain injury, multiple sclerosis, or other disorders—will experience difficulty remembering the context, order, and details of memories. Those with parietal damage often complain that their memories do not appear as vivid and "life-like" compared to their retrieval of memory prior to their brain injury. It turns out that Alzheimer's disease damages all of these brain regions, which is one of the reasons that it causes such devastating memory impairments. We will discuss these and other disorders of episodic memory in more detail in Chapters 13 and 14.

WANT TO KNOW MORE?

Have we whetted your appetite and now you'd like to know more about episodic memory? More about why you remember some things easily and others not at all? More tips to get information into your memory and keep it there? More strategies to retrieve remote memories? More explanations about why forgetting occurs or false memories appear? More techniques to improve your episodic memory, such as associating information and controlling what you remember and forget? All these issues and more will be discussed in detail in Part 2—stay tuned.

But before we continue, what about the patient introduced at the beginning of the chapter and the explanation of Ribot's law? We've saved this part for last because it is an active area of research and there's a bit of controversy about what is the correct answer.

MEMORIES FOR A LIFETIME

Let's consider how you can retain memories over time. Will you remember that breakfast when you learned about John Lennon's death for the rest of your life? If so, how does that happen?

Tag That Memory

The first thing that needs to happen is for your brain to realize that this event of your life is important in some way, and so its memory is worth saving. Perhaps the event is highly emotional, important to you, or distinctive in some other way. Such memories become "tagged" by your brain for long-term storage. Emotional events, for example, release adrenaline and related hormones in your body that help to "tag" the memory as one you should retain. We'll discuss this process of tagging important memories more in Part 2.

Consolidation

Tagged memories are then turned into long-term memories through a process known as *consolidation*. When consolidation occurs, the connections are strengthened between the brain regions related to the sights, sounds, smells, tastes, thoughts, and emotions of the memory episode. Returning to our breakfast example, if that memory becomes consolidated, the sight of the newspaper headlines in your occipital lobe and the sounds of the song *Imagine* in your temporal lobes become linked together, along with the brain activity for the other components of the memory, such as the smell of the onions.

Although much of the consolidation process is still unknown, we know that sleep is critically important (see Chapter 20).

While consolidation can take place when you are awake (particularly if you are resting), the direct linking together of the different components of a memory occurs mainly during sleep. Consolidation can begin soon after an event, but the process continues over many months or even years.

Real Memories . . . or Stories?

So, consolidated memories have their connections strengthened . . . but is the hippocampus still needed to retrieve that memory? Yes and no. Most researchers believe that in order to have that subjective sense of "time-traveling" when you relive a memory, the connection to the hippocampus must still be present in the consolidated memory.[3] Consolidated memories that have lost the connection to the hippocampus become more of a "story" that you remember of what happened to you, rather than a true reliving of the actual event. You may recall both the general outline and quite a lot of facts of what happened during that event of your life, but it isn't quite the same as retrieving a memory in which you can relive the event.

Do you have any childhood memories for events that you retell in roughly the same way each time? Does it no longer feel to you like you're transported back to that past moment when you tell that story? Even if you try, are you unable to see the world from your child-height vantage point, or to bring to mind other sights or sounds or smells that aren't commonly included in your story? While there is no litmus test, if your answer to all these questions is "yes," then you may have a childhood memory that, over time, has lost its connection with the hippocampus.

RIBOT'S LAW EXPLAINED

With the knowledge you have learned in this chapter, you are now ready to understand the basis of Ribot's law and the answer to the question posed by the daughter of the patient at the beginning of this chapter: *How can my father's memory be so good for things that happened 60 years ago when he can't remember what happened yesterday or last month?* We now understand that when the hippocampus is damaged by head trauma, Alzheimer's, or other disorders, there are a number of consequences:

- The formation of new memories will be compromised because of impaired hippocampal binding and indexing.
- Any recent memories that are solely dependent upon the hippocampus will be difficult or impossible to retrieve.
- Some older, consolidated memories, whose components are directly linked together, may be partially independent of the hippocampus and thus can still be retrieved. These older memories, however, will be closer to stories that are remembered than actual episodic autobiographical memories.

* * *

You now understand the basics about how you acquire, store, and retrieve autobiographical memories—memories for the events that make up your life. We will continue to explore autobiographical event memories in Part 2. But next we turn to how you are able to learn, retain, and retrieve knowledge about the world. As we will discuss, it is with this type of memory that the full power of consolidation is realized.

WAYS TO IMPROVE YOUR EPISODIC MEMORY

- Pay attention to your sensations, thoughts, and emotions.
  - Focusing on the sights, sounds, smells, tastes, thoughts, and feelings while you are experiencing them will help you form long-lasting memories.

- Focus on the differences between two similar events if you wish to remember each of them distinctly.
  - To recall each distinctly, concentrate on the distinguishing features of different people, puppies, or parking spots.
- To enhance your retention, review an event after it has concluded.
  - To remember your evening out, think about each aspect of the night as you are traveling home: how you looked in the mirror before you left, the sounds you heard when you opened the door, how others were dressed, the tastes of the food, the faces of the people you met, and the topics you discussed.

5

Semantic memory

What you know

A college professor was referred to the clinic for memory problems. Although she admitted to trouble with names, she reported her memory as "pretty good." She then went on to speak about current events with a fair amount of detail. She was only 63 years old and, at this point in the interview, Andrew was thinking, "Well, perhaps her memory is normal after all." He asked about her other medical problems, and she began to speak about a past surgery. She rolled up her left pants leg and explained that "this one" was done, showing him a long scar across her knee, and then proceeded to roll up her right pants leg, saying that "this one" needed to be done, flexing the right knee and wincing a bit as she did so.

"What do you call that joint?" Andrew asked.

"Oh, I don't know the technical name," she responded.

"What's the ordinary name?"

She shook her head and said, "I don't know."

"It's your knee, right?"

"Knee?" she replied, shaking her head, "What's a knee?"

"You know, it's like your elbow," Andrew said, showing her his own, "except for your leg."

"Elbow, elbow . . . I know the word, but I don't know what it means."

On further questioning it became clear that she had lost the meaning of many words that referred to body parts and articles of clothing.

FACTS AND OTHER THINGS YOU KNOW = YOUR KNOWLEDGE BASE = YOUR SEMANTIC MEMORY

How can this college professor remember news events and what she did last week but not remember what the words "knee" and "elbow" mean? It is, in part, from such individuals that we know there must be a separate memory system that stores our knowledge of the world, including the names we use for things.

We call this system *semantic memory*. The word "semantic" refers to the *meaning* of something and, in fact, some individuals with semantic memory impairment lose not only the words that signify items but also the meaning and use of those items. For example, some patients lose not only the words "fork" and "remote control" but also the meaning of what those items are and their ability to use them, as if they grew up in a culture that did not use forks or remote controls.

Semantic memory constitutes your knowledge of the world that is not related to a specific event that you recall—in other words, unrelated to a particular episodic memory. For example, you probably remember who Queen Victoria and Leonardo da Vinci are, but not where you were and what you were doing when you first learned about them. Similarly, you likely know that the primary colors are red, blue, and yellow, and that if you mix blue and yellow you make green, but not how you know this information. And, of course, you know what to do with forks, screwdrivers, straws, and remote controls even though you probably cannot recall how you learned this information.

ACQUIRING NEW FACTS: BUILDING YOUR SEMANTIC MEMORY

Building new semantic memories is essentially the same thing as learning new facts. Sometimes this means learning information from a textbook, such as who fought in the War of 1812 or what the French word *l'amour* means. Other times it comes from your experience, such as if you hold very still, a parakeet may eat out of your hand, or if you arrive at the cinema to watch the new movie 10 minutes before it starts, it will likely be sold out. As these examples suggest, you need to use your episodic memory to efficiently get information into sematic memory. So, to learn new semantic information, typically the same processes take place as when you are learning new episodic information.

For example, a few days or weeks after you first learn the conjugation of a French verb, you can recall exactly where you sat in the classroom, how the teacher wrote the words on the board, and how she pronounced each one. You can also recall how the sun streamed in through the open window and how you were perspiring slightly on that early September day. Thus, you learned the verb by forming a new episodic memory. Over the next 9 months, however, you proceed to study that verb in your textbook, listen to it being pronounced on videos, and speak it in conversation with classmates. By May, you've studied that verb hundreds of times. You know how to use it perfectly, but no longer recall your initial learning of that verb in the classroom nor the details of your other sessions in which you were studying it. The information has moved from being tied to a specific event to information that is unrelated to any particular episode of your life—it is now part of your semantic memory.

FROM EPISODIC TO SEMANTIC MEMORY

For a memory to move from an event of your life to part of your knowledge base (in other words, from a hippocampally-dependent episodic memory to a semantic memory), two things generally happen in your brain.

Consolidation

One thing that turns events of your life into knowledge is that process of consolidation that we discussed in Chapter 4. For example, the first time you heard the word "lightsaber" was probably when you were watching one of the *Star Wars* movies. Shortly after seeing that movie you might even be able to recall the scene—perhaps the one in which Obi Wan gave a lightsaber to Luke. You can remember the bright blue shimmer it had and the characteristic sounds it made when it was turned on, turned off, and swished through the air. Over time, when you are sleeping, the process of consolidation takes place, directly linking together the word "lightsaber" (stored with your vocabulary in the outer and lower parts of your temporal lobe) with its image (stored with other images in your occipital lobe) and its sounds (stored with other sounds in the upper part of your temporal lobe).

After the memory has been consolidated, if you happen to run into the word, image, or sound of a lightsaber, its other attributes will immediately spring to mind—but you will have lost that personal, autobiographical, time-traveling aspect of the memory back to when you watched that scene in the movie. Note that this doesn't necessarily mean you will have forgotten that scene, just that your experience won't be as vivid or life-like.

Is it a bad thing to lose the episodic nature of your memory for facts? Not at all. If you're helping your friend assemble a piece of furniture and she says, "Pass me the screwdriver," you don't need to be reliving the experience of every prior time you've used a screwdriver, you just need to know what it looks like so you can find it from the array of tools scattered on the floor and hand it to her.

Got the Gist?

Another thing that happens to semantic memories is that they become generalized, such that you are able to discern a variety of different-looking smartphones, car models, can openers, tulips, and tigers even if you have never seen those particular ones before. Together, the hippocampus and the lobes of the brain are, in fact, quite good at extracting the general concept, idea, or gist of a collection of items, and storing that gist away for later retrieval. For example, because of your experience with beach balls, you know the gist of them is that they are filled with air, very light, at least a foot or two in diameter, often brightly colored, and float in water. Your gist of a baseball is very different; it is small enough to be held in your hand, quite hard and solid, heavy for its size, and will sink in water. The gist of your experience with beach balls and baseballs can be consolidated, just like particular features of episodic memories.

This ability to extract and retain the gist of something in your semantic memory is incredibly powerful and quite useful. If you see something that looks like a house cat but has stripes and is about 100 times larger, you don't need to have seen that exact tiger for you to know that it is dangerous and you should stay away. And when your friend returns from the salon you don't say, "Who are you?" (although you have never before seen her with her new hairstyle), but rather, "Nice haircut."

CONSTANTLY UPDATING

This last example, of how you can recognize your friend after her haircut, brings up another important feature of semantic memory, which is that it constantly updates the attributes of things with the latest representations. In other words, even though you may have grown up in the 1970s and developed the concept of "cars" with Ford Pintos and Pontiac Firebirds, your concept of cars has been updated over the last 50 years such that if someone says "car" today you're more likely to think of a Tesla or Toyota Prius.

EPISODIC AND SEMANTIC PEOPLE

Our concepts of individual people generally have both episodic and semantic components. If you think of your family members, you will likely have a number of very specific episodic memories that you can use to travel back in time and relive experiences with them in your mind. You also have a semantic memory concept of each member of your family that is not related to any particular event. This semantic concept includes attributes such as how tall they are, what color their hair is, how they generally dress, and what they like to eat. It also includes their visual appearance, the sound of their voice, and even their mannerisms and how they perform activities.

For example, you might be able to recognize your spouse, children, or friends by the way each of them skis down a slope—very handy when you're trying to meet up with them at the lift. Because people have a semantic component and it is constantly updating, we can now understand why parents cannot usually detect their children growing—the semantic attribute of their height is updated daily. But when your Aunt Marge comes to visit, she notices because—not having seen the children for a year—her semantic image of them is a year out of date. (In fact, Aunt Marge's semantic image may be more than a year out of date, as her image is an average of a number of prior experiences—including when the children were even younger.)

RETRIEVING SEMANTIC KNOWLEDGE

When you are trying to retrieve semantic information, sometimes it comes to mind readily and without effort. In this case what generally happens is that a cue from the environment—perhaps the visual image of the word *"Bahnhof"* on your German vocabulary quiz—activates attributes that are related by their meaning and have been linked together through consolidation, such as the German word for train (*Zug*) and the

English word "station," and you easily write down "train station" on the exam sheet.

At other times the information you are looking for does not spontaneously come to mind. You're sure you know the person's name, vocabulary word, mathematical formula, or biological process but you're drawing a blank. When this happens, your brain's *central executive* needs to use a strategy to find the missing information (see Chapter 3 for more on the central executive). One good strategy is to think about other attributes that you can bring to mind regarding the information you're seeking. For example, you see your friend's face, but this visual image is not automatically bringing up her name. Think about her career, children, hometown, favorite foods, and other information that you can recall about her. It is likely that one of these pieces of information will be linked together with her name, allowing you to retrieve it. We will discuss other retrieval strategies in Chapter 9 (Part 2) and Chapters 22 through 25 (Part 5).

WHERE ARE WORDS IN THE BRAIN?

Now that you know what semantic memory is and how it works, you might be wondering where it is stored in the brain. Hanna and Antonio Damasio, wife-and-husband neurologists who combine their clinical work with neuroscience research, conducted a pair of relevant studies published in 1996 while they were at the University of Iowa. They demonstrated that retrieving words for specific items depends upon the left temporal lobe, including its tip (often called the "temporal pole") just behind your left eye, and its lower and outer extent as it stretches backward toward your occipital lobe in the back of your head.

In the first experiment, they studied over 100 individuals who had strokes in the outer part of their left temporal lobe. They found that those individuals who had strokes in their temporal pole had the most difficulty naming people. Those who had strokes slightly farther back, in the middle of the temporal lobe by the ear, had the most difficulty naming animals. And those who had strokes in the portion of the temporal lobe just behind the ear had the most difficulty naming tools and other manmade objects.

In the second experiment, they used a positron emission tomography (PET) scan to measure brain activity when healthy young individuals were naming either people, animals, or tools. They found that the activity was greatest in the temporal pole when they were naming people, greatest in the back of the temporal lobe when they were naming tools, and more in the middle of the temporal lobe when they were naming animals.

These experiments—along with other work in humans and animals—suggest that not only is your vocabulary stored in your left temporal lobe, but different parts of your temporal lobe are somewhat specialized for remembering different types of words.

WHERE ARE OTHER ATTRIBUTES IN THE BRAIN?

OK, so your words are in the outer part of the left temporal lobe. But what about the image of Cleopatra, the opening sounds of Beethoven's Fifth Symphony, or the taste and texture of an orange wedge as you bite into it? We and most researchers believe that these parts of your knowledge are located close to where these visual, auditory, gustatory, and tactile sensations are formed. Thus, your store of visual images would be in your occipital lobes (which enables vision), your memory of sounds would be in the top part of your temporal lobes (which enables hearing), your memory for tactile sensations would be in your parietal lobes (which enables touch), and so forth. As mentioned earlier in our lightsaber example, if a particular semantic memory has multiple modalities—such as the color, taste, and texture of an orange—the brain representations of these different attributes will be directly connected to each other and to the word "orange" in your temporal lobe, such that you could close your eyes, feel the smooth yet uneven surface of an orange, and immediately have its name, color, and taste spring to mind from your semantic memory.

NORMAL AGING AND SEMANTIC MEMORY

Many older adults have trouble coming up with the names of people and other proper nouns—so many that it is considered part of normal aging. Why do older adults have trouble with names? Although no one is entirely sure and there are several competing theories, it may be due to frontal lobe dysfunction—common in normal aging—that makes retrieval of this semantic information difficult. It is also interesting to note that brain shrinkage in the temporal pole is also so prevalent in older adults that it is considered "normal." Recall that we learned from the Damasios that retrieving the names of people depends upon the proper function of the temporal pole. It is, therefore, at least plausible that healthy older adults experience trouble with names *because* of the shrinkage in the temporal pole. Future research may reveal whether the shrinkage and naming difficulties are truly connected or whether it's just a coincidence. (Why, you may ask, does the temporal pole shrink with normal aging? One speculation is that it might be a side effect of walking upright.)

DISORDERS OF SEMANTIC MEMORY

Now that you know where semantic memory is located in the brain, it should not surprise you to learn that disorders that damage the outer part of the temporal lobes impair semantic memory. Alzheimer's disease is the most common disorder that disrupts semantic memory. This explains why individuals with Alzheimer's disease—in addition to having difficulty remembering recent events with their episodic memory—also have word-finding difficulties. In fact, it is such a common problem in this disease that family members often develop the habit of jumping in with the word their loved one is looking for.

There is also the disorder that our professor had at the beginning of this chapter, the *semantic variant of primary progressive aphasia*. That's a mouthful, but all it really means is that it's slowly *progressive*, the *primary* disorder is with language (*aphasia* means "speechless" in Greek), and *semantic* memory is impaired. Like our professor, these individuals have lost many of the words for everyday people, animals, and things—as if they forgot their primary language. There is also a related disorder called *semantic dementia*. The difference is that although those with the former disorder may have lost the words Kamala Harris, parrot, and cup, if they are shown pictures, they still know that she was the first woman to be vice president, it's a bird that can talk, and it's used for drinking. Those with semantic dementia may not know who Kamala Harris is or what parrots or cups are, as if they grew up in a culture without these people, animals, and things. We'll briefly discuss these disorders in Chapter 13.

Because a lot of other brain disorders can affect the temporal lobes, there are a lot of other causes of semantic memory impairments, including tumors, strokes, and infections such as encephalitis. We'll discuss these disorders in Chapter 14.

WANT TO IMPROVE YOUR MEMORY FOR FACTS?

As mentioned in the beginning of this chapter, you use your episodic memory to learn new facts. In Part 2 you will learn more about what helps—and what hinders—long-term episodic and semantic memories, including memories for facts. And Parts 4 and 5 are entirely devoted to what you can do to remember everything better, from people's names to dates, facts, and formulas. In other words, read on! (And feel free to jump directly to those sections if you wish.)

Below are a few key suggestions that will help you learn new semantic information:

- Form strong episodic memories of the facts you wish to learn.
  - Because semantic memory is based on the information acquired through episodic memory, it is critical to begin with a strong episodic memory.
- Get a good night's sleep.
  - Whether you are trying to remember to remember vocabulary words, history dates, mathematical formulas, or a new programming language, you'll remember information better if you put down your book and allow your brain to consolidate your memories during sleep.
- Study facts in different contexts.
  - Part of what makes semantic memory powerful is that it is knowledge you can pull out and use in a variety of different situations. In order to make your knowledge flexible, study facts in different ways. Cue yourself with a word to recall its definition, and also cue yourself with the definition to recall the word.

6

Collective memory

What we remember together

You're walking with your spouse down a country lane when you come to an old mill. "I just love these old mills with their waterwheels," you say. "It reminds me of the photo we have of the two of us in front of the mill in Pennsylvania when we were planning our wedding."

"Yes," your spouse replies, "except that mill was in New Jersey, not Pennsylvania, and that photo was from the first time you met my parents, not when we were engaged."

"That's right," you say, the memory coming back to you now, as you recall how you went to the mill after meeting your future in-laws, set up your tripod, and took the picture. Returning home, you pull the old picture out and smile. Sure enough, you can see the symbol for the New Jersey Register of Historic Places in front of the mill. But what's that? You look closely—and can clearly see the hand proudly showing the new engagement ring.

It's natural to think about your memories as belonging to you. After all, they are created by *your* brain, reflect *your* past, and help *you* to make decisions about *your* future. But before we close Part 1, we want to challenge you to think about "your" memories a little differently, to reflect that some of their utility

comes from the way they are shared with others, and to consider that they are shaped by those with whom you reminisce.

THE POWER OF SHARED MEMORIES

The prior chapter discussed semantic memory, the set of factual
knowledge you have accumulated over your lifetime. Much of
it is hard-earned knowledge—acquired because you took the
time to read, study, and listen—and, in that sense, it is most
definitely yours. But now consider that much of the power of
this knowledge comes from the fact that it overlaps with the
content in others' memory stores. If you were the only one to
know the meaning of "fork" or "remote control," the knowledge
would be of little use to you. Even in domains of expertise—
where there is utility in holding knowledge that not everyone
has—there must be some foundational shared knowledge that
allows you to understand the problem at hand and to effectively
apply your expertise.

SHARED SCAFFOLDING

Over your lifetime, you not only acquire facts about the world,
but also develop ways to organize that knowledge. Picture a
classroom. You may have quickly brought to mind a rectangular-
shaped room, with a teacher standing at the front and with students sitting quietly at rows of desks facing the front. This image
forms effortlessly, because you have an organized scaffolding or
schema for a typical classroom. Schemas can include information not only about spatial layout but also about the progression
of events. Imagine arriving for your first appointment at a new
doctor's office. Even though you've not been there before, your
schema likely includes details such as first checking in with a
receptionist, filling out forms on a clipboard, and then taking a
seat in a waiting room until you are called. Depending on your
experiences, your schema may include other details, like the

tendency for appointments to run behind schedule or the presence of magazines in the waiting area.

These types of schemas are incredibly helpful. When Elizabeth walks into a new classroom on the first day of the semester, she doesn't need to expend any mental effort to figure out where she should stand. And you don't risk waiting in a doctor's office for hours because you didn't know to tell them you'd arrived.

When There Is No Scaffolding

With the COVID-19 pandemic, we all experienced the discomfort that happens when we are placed in circumstances for which our schemas are incorrect or nonexistent. You might have arrived for a doctor's visit to find that the waiting area was closed. When Elizabeth walked into a classroom that had furniture rearranged to allow for physical distancing, it took her a moment to figure out where she should stand. She also had to work to remember the sanitizing steps that had never previously been part of her getting-ready-for-class schema.

Pushing yourself into situations in which you have no schemas can be an exciting and positive experience, such as when you travel to a part of the world you haven't visited before or take a class on a topic that is entirely new to you. But with the exhilaration comes added mental effort, because you are unable to take as many shortcuts in figuring out what will happen next. Things that might be obvious when you're in familiar territory—how much you should tip after a meal, whether you should drink the water, or how you should prepare for an exam—may suddenly require substantial thought in these novel contexts. Keep in mind that if the first days of a trip feel exhausting or if you doubt your ability to succeed as you begin a new course of study, part of your effort is expended building up the scaffolding that will make the next phase of the trip or the preparation for the next exam easier.

Shared Scaffoldings Shape Individual Memories

Schemas don't just make life easier in the moment. They also shape what content you'll later be able to remember about those moments. It's fairly easy to remember information consistent with your schema (there were magazines in the doctor's office). It can be particularly hard to remember information that is entirely missing from your schema (did you pay when checking in, or at the end of your appointment?). And when information is inconsistent with your schema (the doctor saw you on time), sometimes the surprise can make the detail memorable, but other times, you'll default to the knowledge held in your schema and have an erroneous memory (you may later think the doctor was behind schedule, as usual).

When individuals have similar schemas, similar content will get into their memories and similar content will be left out. So, if you are a superhero fan and you watch a superhero movie in a theater with dozens of other fans, there will be much overlap in what you all remember from the movie. But there can also be informative points of departure: If the movie includes a car chase through the streets of Tokyo, moviegoers who have spent substantial time there may remember the scenes filmed on location in Tokyo much better than those filmed in the studio. Moviegoers who are car aficionados may best remember the moments when a car completed a turn with the tight turning radius it is known for, or when the camera angle highlighted the aerodynamic features of a car's design. If you have no schema for either Tokyo or sports cars, you may remember little about the car chase; you might even omit it from your recall of the movie altogether.

When people remember events together, they also develop similar memory structures for those past events.[1] This means that members of a community who reminisce about events together will build similar schemas, which in turn can lead them to create more similar individual memories for later events. This also means that individuals who are *not* part of those reminiscences can develop different schemas. Sometimes, these differences can be largely irrelevant, but other times, they can radically color how individuals remember and interpret events.

COLLECTIVE MEMORY AND SHARED NARRATIVES

Groups of individuals often share more than just the scaffolding for memories. You can have whole narratives and representations of past events that you share with small groups of individuals or large communities of people, from your family members or roommates to your company, school, congregation, political party, or country. These memories might be representations of events you personally remember, or they might be events that took place before you were born but have been described to you with enough repetition that they have become part of your store of knowledge. These shared event representations are termed *collective memory*, a phrase that aptly captures both their extension to all members of a group and their reliance on gathering together information to preserve it over time.

Wars and Family Feuds

Collective memory at the level of large communities often refers to representations of historical events, such as the narratives regarding a war or the ability to recount a country's leaders. In a series of studies, the psychologists Henry Roediger and Andrew DeSoto have shown that, although these narratives are often shared within a country or generation, there are important divergences across geographical or generational boundaries. For instance, most individuals have a narrative for World War II, even if they were not alive at the time. If you're an American, part of the shared narrative is that you probably consider the attack on Pearl Harbor and D-Day as critical events. But that shared narrative can diverge and splinter in various ways. Many older Americans viewed the bombings of Japan positively (focusing on how they ended the war and spared lives), while most younger Americans viewed them quite negatively (focusing on the death and destruction they caused). Russians remember events not known by many Americans, such as the Battle of Stalingrad, and they refer to the war as the Great Patriotic War rather than World War II. Like individual people, whole countries tend to overestimate their contributions to international efforts, often referred to as "national narcissism." Citizens—whether from Allied or Axis countries—tend to remember their country's contribution to the war as greater than it actually was.[2]

These collective memories are built up through many avenues: books read, lessons learned in school, media coverage of events. But it doesn't require such formal recordkeeping for collective memories to emerge. Something similar often plays out in families through conversation. Your parents and grandparents may have a narrative for the rift that happened between your great-grandmother's side of the family and your great-aunt's side of the family. This narrative may influence how you and your siblings think about family members in your great-aunt's lineage and, whether you are consciously aware of it or not, may influence how you interpret and remember their behaviors in the present day. (She wasn't really sick, she just didn't want to attend the family gathering.) Of course, your great-aunt's side of the family has their own narrative for the rift, one that probably differs in some important ways from the narrative passed down to you—and their narrative probably influences how they interpret and remember your actions. So, without meaning to, we may "take sides" because of the narrative we've internalized even though we didn't directly witness an event. Whether in a family, friendship, or romantic relationship, sometimes an important first step toward moving beyond a conflict is recognizing when there are different narrative beliefs that are held about what happened in the past. Until those are acknowledged, and effort is put into counteracting how those narratives may influence the way that current behaviors are interpreted and remembered, it can be nearly impossible not to bring the baggage of past conflicts into the present.

WORKING TOGETHER TO REMEMBER

You may focus on moments when you are alone as you use your memories—such as when taking an exam or remembering a shopping list—but these situations are usually the exception rather than the rule. Your memories are commonly created and retrieved while you're surrounded by others. Perhaps you are part of a study group, working together to learn vocabulary that will be tested on an upcoming exam. Or you're part of a clinical care team, recounting together the events that precipitated the patient's transfer to your unit. Perhaps you are reminiscing over dinner, enjoying the positive emotions that spring forth as you recount your honeymoon with your spouse. Or maybe you're sharing a memory online, posting photos and making comments with your friends about your weekend spent together. In each case, memory becomes a collaborative venture—and that affects the way that memory works in some interesting ways.

Collaborative Memory

From classrooms to boardrooms, we often work with others to learn information. The support we receive in these collaborative environments can be essential to our ability to learn. Collaborative learning can provide a powerful way to increase critical thinking skills and can help you move past sticking points in your ability to learn information.[3] So, whether you're a student struggling to make sense of the material presented in class or part of a clinical care team trying to understand a patient's symptoms, it will help you to collaborate with others.

If your goal is not to *understand* material but only to improve how much and how well you can *commit* something to memory, collaborating with others will not always help you achieve that goal. Collaborating with others does not always bring about memory benefits and, in fact, there can be some important downsides.[4] While you collaborate with others, you will encode and store some of these details into your own memory, and the group's efforts may help you stay more motivated, and in these ways, you can benefit from the collaboration. But there also can be downsides. Perhaps counterintuitively, collaboration can make it harder for you to memorize information or to retrieve previously learned details from memory than if you worked on your own. It also can be hard to distinguish the memory of the group from your individual memory. You might leave a study group feeling great about how many historical facts you know, only to realize (as you begin the exam) that some of that content was only represented in others' brains—and not in yours. Another problem is that if someone in the group is wrong, the errors can also be transmitted to others in the group. So, if you're a student who needs to memorize vocabulary, or a consultant on a team trying to learn content for a presentation that you—and you alone—will be giving, be sure the pros outweigh the cons before making those memory tasks a collaborative effort.

Reminiscing

We often spend time with others to retrieve shared memories, not because we need to perfectly recreate a past event, but because of the positive emotions and feelings of social connectedness that result from bringing such events to mind. Memories can provide a powerful social glue, making you feel connected with people even if you haven't seen them in some time. Reminiscing can boost your mood, not only because of this social connectedness but also because the memories themselves can be rewarding. Megan Speer, Jamil Bhanji, and Mauricio Delgado at Rutgers University revealed that reflecting on a positive past event activates reward circuitry in the brain. In fact, the positive memories were so rewarding that, when they gave participants a choice between retrieving a positive memory or receiving a small financial reward, participants were willing to forgo money in order to reminisce about the positive moments from their past![5]

DID IT HAPPEN TO ME?

Sometimes the narratives you share with others can blur the lines between what is a memory of your own personal past and what is a memory another has shared with you. Disputes over what-happened-to-whom are relatively common among siblings, especially among twins. In one study, 20 sets of twins were shown cue words and asked to recall a memory that came to mind from their personal past. Fourteen of the twin pairs produced at least one overlapping memory; that is, they each reported the same memory in response to the cue word, claiming the event had happened to them and not their twin.[6] For instance, one set of 21-year-old twins both remembered that, when they were 5, they were pushed off their bicycle by their cousin. Another set of twins, now 56, both remembered that when they were 13 they fell off a tractor and sprained their wrist. These memories were vivid and—interestingly—many were memories that the siblings did not know were in dispute until that experiment; they had lived their lives believing the event had happened to them, with no reason to doubt the memory.

In general, we trust the memories of people we're close to, allowing them to fill in the gaps of our own memories. In one study, either couples or strangers were asked to separately watch a short film and then discuss the details. Unbeknownst to them, they had watched slightly different versions of the film. When one person generated a detail, the other sometimes accepted it as true, even though it had not appeared in their version of the film. This acceptance of incorrect details happened at a much higher rate among the couples than it did among the strangers.[7] As in the story at the start of the chapter, when it's someone you're close to, someone you trust, you not only are likely to use their knowledge to fill in the gaps of your own memories, but you may also accept their memories as accurate representations of your past, such that you'll incorporate their—sometimes incorrect—recollections into your own. In a fundamental way, the way you remember your life is influenced by the memories of others.

WHERE DO YOUR MEMORIES END AND OUR MEMORIES BEGIN?

As you read on in this book, we hope you'll keep this shared memory perspective in mind. From here on out, we'll return to talking about your memories, and remembering your past. But now you know that, because your memories exist in the context of others' memories, the way you represent your past is going to be shaped not only by the neural patterns within your brain but by the broader contexts and societal narratives that mold those patterns, and by the memories that others have shared with you.

THE BENEFITS AND DRAWBACKS OF COLLECTIVE MEMORY

- When you're in unfamiliar territory without shared scaffoldings or schemas to guide you, it may take you a bit longer to get the hang of things before you begin to feel comfortable.
  - So, whether you're traveling, studying a new subject, or learning a new hobby, stick with it and you'll get there.

- Don't be surprised if you and a friend remember different aspects of a shared experience if your background, knowledge, and expertise is different.
  - Beliefs and interpretations of what happened in the past will frequently differ across people, families, organizations, and cultures.
- There are benefits—and drawbacks—to remembering information together while working or studying.
  - Critical thinking skills often increase as you learn from others how to get past sticking points and problem areas you may have faced alone.
  - Be careful, however, of studying for exams or preparing for presentations in a group if you—and you alone—will be required to recall all of the information. Otherwise, although the group as a whole might know all the needed content, you as an individual may not have learned it all, and you might have incorporated some inaccurate information as well.
  - We recommend that you study both in groups and by yourself. This way you get the best of both approaches.
- Reminiscing with family, friends, and colleagues can boost your mood and help you feel connected with people even if you haven't seen them in a long time.
- You are likely to fill in the gaps of your own memories with memories of someone you trust.
  - Often this leads to more complete and accurate memories—but sometimes this leads to the incorporation of false and incorrect information into your memory.

Part 2

MAKING MEMORIES

7

Do you need to try to remember?

You pull out of your driveway and turn onto the main street. Your windshield wipers are racing to keep pace with the rain. You suddenly wonder: Did I close the garage door? You know your garage floods in the rain, and so you are usually careful to close the door. Yet, as you search your memory, you draw a blank. You can't remember pressing the button to close the door, and you don't remember seeing it close. The rain is beating harder against the windshield. You sigh, and turn toward home to check. As you approach your house, you see the garage door is closed.

You've probably had many moments like these, when you performed some action yet have no memory of doing so, as if the memory were never created. You now know from Part 1 that this is a problem creating an *episodic memory*[1,2]—such that you cannot consciously bring to mind a specific occurrence from your past. Let's find out why this forgetting occurs—and how to remember these moments better.

EPISODIC MEMORY NEEDS ATTENTION

Lapses in memory usually arise because you weren't paying attention. If you think back to our discussion of sensory memory in Chapter 3, you may recall that when you pay attention, you move visual, auditory, and other sensory information into working memory, where you can keep the information active. If you continue to attend to the information in working memory, it is then ushered into long-term episodic memory. Sounds simple, right? Just pay attention and you'll remember information.

The problem is that we don't pay attention to most information in our environment. Try to imagine what a penny looks like: Not just its color, size, or shape, but its details, too. Whose face is profiled, and in which direction? What is written on the front and back, and where is the text positioned? If you find this surprisingly hard, you're not alone. Even at a time when pennies were spent and received more commonly than they are today, Americans were quite poor at selecting the real penny from foils that had rearrangements or errors in the features.[3] You may think you know what a penny looks like, but unless you are a coin collector, you usually only pay attention to its superficial features. You can identify a penny based on its size and color alone and so don't need to focus on the other details. That means that—despite all the times that you looked at a penny—those details weren't attended to and so they didn't make it into your memory.

INTENTION GUIDES EFFORT

When you're trying to remember something—in other words, when you're intentionally creating a memory—you are more likely to focus your attention on the to-be-remembered content. When learning someone's name, you know you should listen carefully as they pronounce it. In class, you know you should be attentive as the teacher speaks and as you review your textbook. This *intent* to remember can help you weed out distractions and stay focused on the information you seek to retain.

A basic principle of memory is that if we want to form a long-term memory, one that we will have conscious access to weeks or months later, we must devote *effort* to processing the information that will make up that memory. It's not enough to just notice the information. Our eyes can scan a textbook page for a long time, but if we're not expending the effort to thoroughly understand the material and thoughtfully consider the words as we read them on the page, a durable memory is unlikely to be formed.

FIND ORGANIZATION AND MEANING

Often, the effort we exert centers around finding organization and meaning in information.

Try to remember the following words:

---

organization, try, information, often, structure, it, memory, to, giving, content, has, remember, when, little, fails

---

How many of those 15 words could you remember?
Now, try to remember these words:

To remember information, try giving it organization.
When content has little structure, memory often fails.

How many of those 15 words could you remember?

The 15 words are, of course, the same. But you most likely remembered more of the words when they were organized into meaningful sentences than when they were assembled randomly. Organization provides the scaffolding for memory,[4] and the intent to learn usually prioritizes your efforts to organize incoming information. If you attend a conference with the goal of later sharing what you've learned with your coworkers, you are likely to take notes that are organized around the key con-cepts you want to retain and share. If you sit down to study for an exam, you (hopefully) first take a moment to sort through your notes and remind yourself of the big concepts that will be tested.

Of course, even with the intent to learn, that doesn't mean you will automatically be perfect in executing your plans to attend to and organize the material. When exam time looms, you may skip over the organizing step and just frantically re-read por-tions of your notes in the hopes that something "sticks." And we certainly all experience lapses in attention: those moments when you catch yourself daydreaming in a meeting, or realize you weren't listening as someone introduced themselves. When those lapses arise, memory suffers. Simply having the intention to remember isn't enough; only if that intention is backed up by attention and effort can we effectively get content into memory.

DON'T MULTITASK

No matter how good you may think you are at multitasking, when your attention is divided across multiple tasks, your memory suffers.[5] This is such a simple statement, but most of us think that it applies to other people—not to us. The bottom line is that it is true, and it applies to all of us.

If you're messaging with your friends while trying to study, you won't remember the material as well as you could have. If email previews are flashing across your computer while you're preparing for your presentation, you won't be as prepared. And if your partner is speaking to you while you have one eye on the big game, you won't remember half of what they were saying.

LEARNING WITHOUT INTENT

Just as the intent to remember doesn't guarantee that a mem-ory will be formed, *not* having the intent to remember doesn't mean that a memory *won't* be formed. You may marvel at the seemingly trivial details you remember from past events or the arsenal of pop culture knowledge you've amassed.

Memories can be formed *incidentally* through our usual interactions with the world. Although you surely don't spend your holiday dinners or celebrations with friends focused on remembering every moment, you probably have long-lasting memories of many of those events. In large part that's because what you do naturally is exactly what's needed to form a memory on these occasions. You listen closely to a friend's story— not to memorize its content, but because you care about what is happening in their life; nonetheless, as a result of your focused attention and your efforts to understand what happened to them, you are likely to create a lasting memory.

GOALS GUIDE THE CONSTRUCTION OF A MEMORY

So, what you attend to and put effort into determines what you will remember. This means that it is your *goals* as you process events that will affect what information is placed into your memory. If your primary goal isn't to remember the content for later, then whatever other goal you have at the moment will affect what you remember.

Imagine being at a brunch with coworkers as a jazz band performs. You are relatively new to the company, and so you are focused on the interpersonal dynamics at the table and at getting to know your colleagues better. One of your coworkers chose this restaurant because she is considering hiring the band for an upcoming office event. Because of your different goals during the meal, you and your coworker are likely to leave with different memories of the event: You are likely to remember the conversation topics and personal tidbits shared by your colleagues, while your coworker is likely to have much better memory for the songs the band played and others' reactions to their sets.

Sometimes, as in the jazz brunch example, your goals are clear and so it may be easy to understand why you remember some features and not others. At other times, however, your goals are less clear or fixed. For example, at a dinner with extended family, you may shift between wanting to reminisce, trying to steer conversation away from potentially controversial topics, and simply enjoying the food. You may weave between these goals, often without being aware of it. As a result, there may be some portions of the time—perhaps when you were focused on savoring that last bite of pie—when you have little memory for what else was going on in the room. That may explain why everyone else remembers the joke that Aunt Marge told over dessert while you have no memory of it.

VARIABILITY IN MEMORY

No two people will approach an event with exactly the same goals or perspective. This variability makes it hard to predict which aspects someone might remember from an event, and it also is one reason why two people can experience the same event yet remember completely different details. Imagine three eyewitnesses standing on a sidewalk at the time of a hit-and-run accident, each with a clear view of the intersection. All had similar views and similar time to process what was happening, but that doesn't mean that all will create similar memories of the event. The first eyewitness may have been lost in thought until hearing the noise of the crash; by that time, the offending car may have already sped out of sight. The second eyewitness may have noticed the speeding car as it approached the intersection, realized that an accident was about to happen, and may have even tried to remember the make of the car and its license plate. The third eyewitness may have been completely focused on whether anyone was hurt and planning their next action—Should I call 911? Where is my phone?—and may have not paid any attention to the details of the vehicles. Knowing someone's vantage point (and the time they have to process an event) is certainly helpful in determining the likelihood they will remember certain aspects of it, but it isn't sufficient for predicting what they might realistically be *expected* to remember in, for example, a court of law.

WHEN EFFORT TO REMEMBER DOESN'T HELP

Sometimes when you're trying hard to learn something, you may feel so anxious about getting the information into your memory—and fearful that you may not succeed—that it creates considerable anxiety. This anxiety may be so distracting such that it actually diminishes your ability to learn. This can be particularly true if you've experienced failures in the same area before (such as difficulty with math) or if you often struggle with memory in a particular way (such as believing yourself to be "bad with names"). Even simply thinking of a task as a "test of memory" can sometimes lead to worse performance. In one experiment, older adults performed more poorly on a "memory test" than they did on the same task framed as a different activity.[6] Thus, while it's usually beneficial to have the goal of remembering information, there can be some instances when you want to reframe that goal to another one that will keep you fully focused on processing the information—but in a less anxiety-provoking way!

SUCCEEDING AT REMEMBERING

You can now better understand why sometimes, no lasting memory forms. In the example we began the chapter with, your attention was probably focused on navigating out of the driveway in the rain, not on pressing the garage-close button or watching the door close. It's no wonder, then, that moments later you had no memory of closing the door. You may even find yourself without a memory for the story at the start of the chapter, for similar reasons: Perhaps you glossed over the italicized portion of text, not paying it much attention; or perhaps you read it, but never gave it another thought as you read to this point in the chapter. Without that additional effort, a durable memory for the story was never created.

You are now ready to leverage this and the other knowledge you learned in this chapter to help you remember better. Consciously trying to remember can be a powerful way to bring your efforts into alignment with your goals of retaining information. But it isn't the only way to succeed in forming a memory. You will succeed whenever your goals lead you to exert effort toward processing the information. This also means that, by adjusting your goals, you can change what you remember from an event.

To usher the content you want into memory, you'll want to:

- **Avoid distraction—don't multitask!** You want your brain's resources focused on what you hope to remember. Memory suffers when attention is divided.
  - Turn off the podcast and close down your browser tabs. No matter how good you think you are at multitasking, you won't retain as much information if you're splitting your attention between the information you're trying to learn and any other type of content.
  - Put your phone on do-not-disturb and out of sight. Just having your phone *nearby* can serve as a distractor. Even if you never look at it, having the goal of monitoring it for incoming messages and texts may compete with your goal of attending to the content you hope to remember.
- **Align your in-the-moment goals with your memory goals.** What you remember from an event is going to be tied to how you processed the event as it unfolded.
  - If you're interviewing for a job, you may be more focused on making a good impression than on remembering the details of your conversations. But if you plan to write thank-you notes to

those with whom you met, you'll want to keep that secondary goal in mind so that you have some specific content to refer to in each note.

- o If you take the time to savor the happy moments from your relative's fifth birthday party, you will give yourself the best chance of remembering that joy for years to come. Try to appreciate the time spent with him even if you're carrying out mundane duties with him, like setting the table. You may, in fact, get more enjoyment out of those moments as they occur—and you'll likely reap benefits again later when your memory is filled with moments of time spent together.

- **If your goal of remembering is creating anxiety, reframe your goal.** Anxiety can be a source of distraction; it can cause you to ruminate on past memory failures and other unpleasant thoughts rather than being attuned to the information present right now.
  - o For example, when someone introduces themselves, your mind may wander to the last time you failed to learn someone's name— rather than listening carefully to them saying their name now!
  - o If you realize that your anxiety about learning information is getting in your way, a good strategy can be to think of an alternate goal that still facilitates paying close attention. For instance, challenge yourself to make a connection with every name you are told: *She shares my aunt's middle name. He has the same initials as my favorite author.* Not only will you have to pay close attention to each name, but the connections will help you in remembering them. (More on remembering names in Chapter 24.) Most importantly, now it's not a "memory task," but a fun game. See how creative you can be in changing and reframing whatever memory task is stressing you out.

8

Get it into your memory—and keep it there

You worked into the wee hours of the morning on the report for the committee. You rehearsed what you would say as you created each page of the presentation booklet, committing facts and figures to memory. When your head finally hit the pillow, you were feeling good about the presentation, even if you wouldn't get much sleep. A few hours later, you are in the conference room. Your first moments of the presentation go smoothly. Then, you ask everyone to flip to page 3 and, as you stare at the charts, you cannot remember why you chose to display this information. Why did you decide to show these figures? What were you intending to say?

Have you experienced a moment like this one, when you spent time preparing—feeling confident that you memorized the information—yet, when the critical moment arrives, you can't remember what you were going to say? In this chapter we'll examine some of the reasons why the process of keeping information in your memory can go awry.

THE MEMORY CYCLE

To understand these types of errors, we first need to understand how you convert the sights, sounds, smells, thoughts, and feelings that you are currently experiencing into a memory that you will be able to recall in the future.

Long-term episodic memory consists of three phases. First, to have a memory, your brain must take information that exists *right now*—the name you are being told or your thoughts about how you will narrate your presentation—and convert that information to a format that can be stored in your brain. As we mentioned in Chapter 4, this is *encoding*—turning an event into a "neural code." Imagine encoding as building a structure out of blocks that models the current moment of time. That sounds good, but without further action to stick the blocks together, this structure will fall apart and the neural code will be lost. The *long* in long-term memory requires that your brain actively works to hold on to that content. Thus, the second phase of memory is *storage*. The third stage of memory is *retrieval*, when you reconstruct the structure out of its building blocks, thereby allowing you to re-access parts of a prior moment in time (more on this in Chapter 9).

While you might think about retrieval as the end point of a memory, retrieval is also a starting point. When you retrieve a memory, you are actually bringing a past moment into the present. Although the event happened in the past, your reflections on that event are happening *right now* and, as a result, these reflections can automatically restart the memory cycle. In other words, every retrieval is also an opportunity to re-encode that memory anew. Thus, as you retrieve a memory and, by so doing, rebuild the memory structure out of blocks, the "design" decisions you make— which portions of the structure you embellish, which you diminish, and which you leave out entirely—can affect how information is *re-encoded* into memory (see Figure 8.1). As

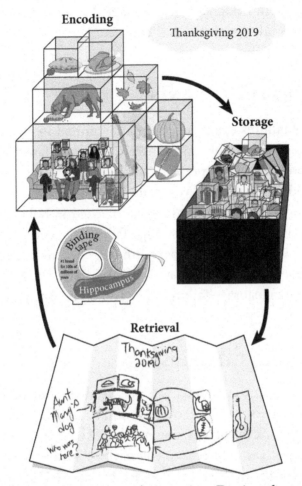

Figure 8.1. The memory cycle in action. During the encoding of an event, different elements of that experience are assembled into a coherent memory structure, with the hippocampus acting as the binding tape. Those elements are then stored, with the hippocampus holding on to the blueprints for how to reassemble them. At retrieval, the blueprints are used to reconstruct the memory structure, with the hippocampus again serving as the tape that binds the elements together.

we will see in Chapter 12, this cyclical re-encoding process can subtly alter or even radically change a memory—and can do so permanently.

FAILURES IN THE CYCLE

Memory failures can result from a disruption in any of these phases of the memory cycle. You could have failed to build and represent your experience in a way that can be stored—an encoding failure. Or you could have built the experience, but without the structural integrity needed to hold on to the information over time—a storage failure. Or you could have stored the knowledge yet have difficulty reconstructing it at the moment it is needed—a retrieval failure. We'll focus on encoding and storage failures now, and on retrieval failures in Chapter 9.

ENCODING FAILURES

Encoding failures abound. You may read the same sentences of your textbook over and over, yet still be unable to look away and recite back the details. You may be asked to describe someone you just saw and realize you have no idea about some of their key features: Were they wearing glasses? How long was their hair?

Think back to the examples from the prior chapter: how you could not remember whether you closed the garage door, or how little any of us remember about a penny's details. These represent encoding failures—or at least encoding choices. It turns out that your brain is quite efficient at pulling in the *gist*—the general content or theme of information.[1] You can quickly encode that you're looking at a person who is a woman, taller than you, with dark hair. But it's a more demanding process for your brain to pull in all the details, to build the representation of the person to include specifics such as the shape of her glasses or the length of her hair. Without substantial effort, those details won't be included in the memory.

FOCUS ATTENTION, ORGANIZE, UNDERSTAND, RELATE

To avoid encoding failures and minimize forgetting, try FOUR things:

Focus attention
Organize
Understand
Relate.

First, **Focus**: Pay attention to the information you are trying to remember, which will devote your brain's resources to its processing. As discussed in Chapter 7, avoid distractions so that you can focus your attention on the to-be-remembered content.

Second, **Organize**: Organizing information is one good way to decrease the demands placed on the brain during encoding. Sometimes, these differences can be largely irrelevant, but other times, they can radically color how individuals remember and interpret an event. Imagine trying to memorize a phone number by its 10 separate digits: 5-0-5-2-1-4-1-0-3-1; that's 10 things to remember—too much for most people. As we mentioned in Chapter 3, you can make it easier on yourself by *chunking* it into the more familiar 505-214-1031. This is a bit easier, but it will also take a lot of rehearsal, and you might still make some mistakes, such as reversing the order of some numbers. Next, imagine the sets of digits as dates (May 5th, February 14th, October 31st). Now you have only three chunks of information to remember, the three dates. It's as if, instead of trying to construct a memory out of 10 separate blocks, one for each digit, you can now construct the same memory from just three blocks because you've stuck a bunch of the little blocks together—making the whole structure much easier to encode.

It might take some time and creativity to find the patterns in a phone number that would be helpful for memorizing it, but even those efforts will make it more likely that you can encode the number into your memory without errors.

Third, **Understand**: Make sense of what you are trying to remember. Understanding information is different than simply spending time rehearsing it. No matter how many times you read about the Krebs cycle in your biology textbook, you are unlikely to encode the cycle into memory unless you're trying to understand what you are reading.

Fourth, **Relate**: Connect the information to what you already know, or to things important to you. We acquire new knowledge by linking it to what we already understand. Without the foundational knowledge in place, new learning is more difficult. Imagine trying to learn long division without having already mastered addition and subtraction. The knowledge you start with provides a scaffolding that can allow you to learn new information with less effort. For example, once you have memorized the major bones in the body, it is much easier to learn the muscles that move them, and then the arteries that nourish the muscles.

Sometimes, the links between your existing concepts or events and the new information you are trying to remember may occur to you quickly and easily. In the phone-number example, you might have noticed that May 5th is Cinco de Mayo, February 14th is Valentine's Day, and October 31st is Halloween. Those connections to your existing knowledge will make this information even easier to encode into memory—like using building blocks that you've already stuck together. Sometimes you may need to work harder to find the links, but the more effort you put into finding those connections, the more likely you will successfully encode the content into memory.

Part of the power of relating new information to our prior knowledge is that it can help us to organize the new

information and give it meaning. Chess experts can look at a
board and quickly retain a memory for where the pieces are, in
part because each placement has meaning (the queen is being
threatened, checkmate in three moves) and in part because
they can chunk the board into smaller units so they don't need
to memorize each piece separately.[2] When a novice looks at the
board, they only see the separate pieces; they don't have the
knowledge to recognize meaningful patterns and chunk the
pieces together. (Consistent with this idea, when chess experts
are shown a board with the pieces distributed randomly, without placements that could have occurred through playing, they
don't show the same benefits in remembering the pieces on the
board.)

ENCODED, BUT FORGOTTEN

Sometimes, it's clear that you encoded a memory. But mere
hours later, it's as if the memory has vanished. As you finish
studying and close your textbook, you can confidently summarize the Krebs cycle. A few hours later, to your horror, you
cannot recognize any of the details on the multiple-choice test.
This type of memory error, like the one we began the chapter
with, suggests a storage failure. The memory was encoded and
briefly existed, yet the content was not maintained.

At the turn of the 20th century, the fact that we forget was one
of the first principles of memory to be discovered and system-
atically studied by the German scientist Hermann Ebbinghaus.
Recently-learned information follows a predictable "forgetting curve," with much information lost soon after learning.[3]
Indeed, extensive forgetting is the norm. Think about everything you did so far today that you can recall easily—what you
ate for breakfast, which mug you drank your coffee from, where
you found this book, and when you picked it up and continued reading. How many of those details will you remember
tomorrow? A week from tomorrow? Next month? Most likely,

you will recall very few of these details after a few days. Clearly the details were encoded—you can remember them now, even though those moments are in the past—but it's unlikely that you will store them in a durable manner. Memories are usually transient,[4] and only a select few will transition from being available moments after an event has occurred to being available days, weeks, or months later.

Over time, the content we store within a memory will also shift. In the minutes and hours after an event, you are likely to retain a reasonable number of details. Soon after a phone call with your cousin, you will likely remember the tone of their voice, the range of topics discussed, and many specific phrases the two of you used. A few days later, however, while you are likely to recall that the phone call happened, you are unlikely to remember most of these details. As time passes, our memories shift from storing the specifics of what happened to storing the *gist* of the event—its general outline or its meaning to us. This is one reason why our memories can, quite literally, become less vivid over time.[5]

MAKING STORAGE HAPPEN

After an event has occurred, additional changes arise in the brain to ensure that the neural code of the event remains. Storage isn't just something that happens automatically; there are active processes that keep us from forgetting important information. Some of these changes happen soon after we experience an event, resulting in lasting changes in the strength of connections between brain cells. Others unfold over longer periods of time, resulting in widespread changes across a vast network of brain regions.

Some of these active storage processes occur optimally while we are sleeping. That's right—your brain isn't "resting" while you sleep; your brain is actually highly active (a point we'll return to in Chapter 20). The sleeping brain is also active in fundamentally different ways than it can be when you're awake and actively processing the world around you. When distanced from the input of the surrounding world, your brain can go through the important work of sorting through the information encountered during the waking day and keeping the important memories so they are accessible in the future. Sometimes, as in the example at the outset of the chapter, too little sleep can contribute to storage failures by preventing the brain from having the neurobiological environment needed to stabilize the neural code of an event into a long-lasting memory.

PRIORITIZING THE RIGHT CONTENT

How does your brain know which memories to keep? In other words, what makes a memory important to remember? Many of the clues the brain uses to figure out what is important are present as an event is initially being experienced. And the good news is that there are many ways you can help guide your brain to prioritize which memories to keep!

Emotional Content

Your brain relies on your body's responses to experienced events as one of the clues to figuring out whether something is important to you. Did your heart skip a beat when your child called you to announce their engagement? Did you feel your palms sweating as you walked to the front of the room to begin a presentation? The bodily systems that cause you to have these reactions to emotional or stressful events can simultaneously *tag* the ongoing event as one that is of importance.[6] Emotion and stress are designed to help us focus on the parts of our environment that demand our attention *right now*, weeding out other distractions. Later, our brain tends to prioritize the storage of those tagged events.

Even if the information may not be intrinsically emotional, you can often give information emotion by thinking deeply about what your own, personal, emotional reaction to the information would be if it were happening to you. If you're reading about the details of a historical battle or a political campaign, think about the emotions you would feel if you were in the thick of it when the flak was flying fiercely.

Distinctive Content

Content that is surprising or *distinctive*—standing out from other information in some way—can also be prioritized for storage, even if it doesn't elicit a bodily response.[7] Sometimes, that distinctiveness can be thought of as a property of the content. Swear words are conceptually distinctive because of their meaning and their relative taboo (at least in polite society). Textbooks use formatting like **bolding** and underlining to make the information perceptually distinctive—you are more likely to remember content that stands out from other information on the page. Other times, distinctiveness depends upon the context. A snake is often distinctive, but not if you're at the zoo in the reptile house.

To aid your memory, you can find ways to make otherwise ordinary information more distinctive. Highlighting text is one method to achieve perceptual distinctiveness, and it can provide benefits to memory compared to passively reading the material. But do so in moderation—it is no longer distinctive if you've highlighted the whole page. Saying some content aloud can also make it more distinctive. Again, this doesn't work if you say *everything* aloud, but if there are key concepts that you want to commit to memory, or certain takeaway messages that you want to be sure to remember in a presentation, saying them aloud can help to commit them to memory and keep them there.[8] So, as you continue reading this book, perhaps you'll be inspired to highlight some phrases or say aloud an interesting

point that you hope to retain in memory long after you've finished the book. (And if you're specifically trying to learn material in depth, look to Chapter 23 for even more effective ways of
studying material than highlighting.)

Involve the Senses

Another way you can make information stand out is by linking
it to your senses. Give information musicality: Create a jingle
to help you remember the information, or notice the rhyth-
micity of the syllables in someone's name. Construct a mental image: Imagine what someone's name would look like in
neon letters. Rather than trying to memorize that you parked
on level 3H by repeating it over and over, think about writing
a huge letter **H** on a sign, and notice the three brush strokes
you took to form the letter. Or think of three smelly **H**yenas
sitting in your car. The more sensory dimensions you can give
to a memory, the greater the likelihood you will create a lasting
memory trace.

Important to You

Your memories are importantly linked to your self-concept—
after all, your memory is about what happened to *you* in the
past—and therefore information that you can relate to yourself
is more likely to be remembered. We often struggle to learn
information when we can't imagine how it intersects with
our life.

Perhaps you're trying to memorize a series of historical events
and you can't see why you should need to know this information. Figure out ways to make the information relevant to you.
Imagine you are planning a visit to this country, and spend time
thinking about how the historical chain of events you're learning shaped it into the country it is today. Although it may seem
like these efforts are taking time away from your studying, in
reality, by making the information relevant to something you

care about, you will likely find it easier to hold on to the content. So, whether you're trying to understand a chapter in your biochemistry textbook or working to memorize the names of the people you will meet at an upcoming social event, try linking the content to something important to you.

Remember the FOUR Principles

Other cues to importance come from the same processes that we've already talked about earlier in this chapter as benefiting encoding:

Focus attention on the new information.
Organize the content.
Understand its meaning.
Relate the new information to your existing knowledge.

By doing these things you will increase the likelihood that you will initially encode a memory and also that your brain will successfully store it.

FORGETTING ISN'T ALWAYS BAD

Do you wish you could simply take a pill and have the superpower to remember everything? Given the extensive marketing of so-called memory-enhancing vitamins, herbs, supplements, and nutritional drinks, you might think that if such a pill really existed, you should jump at the chance to take it. But while it is easy to think of forgetting as a "glitch," and to imagine the ideal memory system as one that would retain all details, there turn out to be important benefits to forgetting. In fact, just like storage, forgetting is both an active process some of the time and also one that is essential for memory to serve its purpose.[9]

To understand why a memory system that forgets might be more beneficial than one that stores everything, we need to consider why you benefit from memory at all. It may seem obvious that you have memory so that you can know what happened to you in the past. But then again, how useful is it for you to be able to revisit some past moment in time?

MEMORY FOR THE FUTURE

In Lewis Carroll's *Through the Looking Glass,* there's a terrific exchange between Alice and the Queen, where the Queen states, "It's a poor sort of memory that only works backwards." It was an insightful statement that Carroll wrote 150 years ago. Although we tend to think of memory as the ability to hold on to the past, the actual benefits of memory come from its power to allow us to make sense of the *present moment* and to creatively, flexibly plan for the *future.*[10]

Individuals with amnesia, such as Henry described in Chapter 1, not only can't remember what happened to them yesterday or last year, but they also have difficulty imagining what will happen to them tomorrow or next year. If we don't have any episodic memories of past events, then we have nothing to use to help us imagine possible future scenarios. It is because our minds are replete with memories that we can imagine and plan for future events. Even if you've never departed from a particular airport before, you can estimate how much time you need to clear security and reach your gate because you remember approximately how long it took in all the other airports you have departed from. Your gist memories from those prior events give you the information you need to make a wise decision.

Let's dive into this example and consider the content you need to remember to help you make decisions about a future, yet-to-be-experienced scenario. When trying to decide when to leave for the airport, it would be quite inefficient for you to have to sift through your memory for every past airport you've been in, recalling all the details such as gate numbers, flight times, number of people in the security line, and the color of the flight attendants' uniforms. You don't need any of those details to guide your decision. There will not be exactly the same number of people in the security line as the last time you were at an airport (and even if there were, the time they take wouldn't be the same). Rather than getting bogged down in those details, you need a system that enables you to quickly abstract a representation—a schema—of a "generic airport" that is built from your prior experiences but is unlike any particular event you've experienced before.

Forgetting allows us to more easily form abstracted representations; forgetting forces you to quickly—and effortlessly—"see the forest for the trees" because the details of the trees are gone. This loss of details can also make it easier for you to appreciate the interconnections and similarities between prior places and events: how most airports' security lines are set up similarly, how departure gates are numbered, and other features that airports share. As the high-resolution details of events are lost, similar events begin to resemble one another more. So, although there are some benefits to remembering most of your past, there also can be pitfalls to having a memory system that doesn't prioritize forgetting.

HOW NOT TO FORGET

Although forgetting isn't always a bad thing, there are, of course, many times when you've devoted substantial effort to getting details into your memory and you'd like to keep them there. None of us want to end up in the situation described at the start of this chapter—fumbling over a presentation because we've forgotten key points that we intended to communicate.

So, how do we keep from forgetting content that we want to retain?

- Use effort to help you learn and remember the FOUR principles of learning.
  - **Focus** attention on the content you want to remember.

- If you find your attention drifting, direct it back to the material or experience you wish to remember.
- Focus on what your friend is telling you, and try to ignore everything else.
- Help yourself to stay alert by sitting up straight in class.
- And make sure you get enough sleep!
  - ○ **Organize** the material in ways that it will be easier to remember.
    - Before trying to memorize your notes, spend a few moments organizing them into categories or groups that will be easier to remember. Do the same thing with each of the groups, to make them organized as well.
    - Chunk a credit card number that you're trying to commit to memory into a series of dates or scores in basketball games.
    - If you're trying to relearn the names of all your old high school friends for your upcoming reunion, try to remember them by the different groups or social circles that you knew them (glee club, soccer team, math class, etc.).
  - ○ **Understand** what you want to remember.
    - If you're studying material, make sure you understand the frameworks, concepts, and details you're trying to learn.
    - If you're living through a moment you hope to remember, think about the meaning of what is happening around you.
  - ○ **Relate** the information to things you already know, or topics you care about.
    - Trying to memorize an address? Turn the number, street, and town into three concepts that you're familiar with. For example, for 42 Maple Street, Cooperstown, think of Jackie Robinson's jersey number, the large maple tree in the park across the street, and "barrel-making town" (if you happen to know that coopers are people trained to make barrels).
    - Trying to learn a new computer program or smartphone application? Think about how the electronic steps might be analogous to things you're more familiar with, such as moving paper or other physical objects around and manipulating them.
- Make information stand out.
  - ○ Imbue it with emotion.

- Don't just read the historical facts on the page; think about how it would have felt to live through those times.
- Feel the fear, doubt, grief, or triumph of the people in that news story you want to remember to tell your friend.
  ○ Make it distinctive.
    - Say a person's name aloud.
    - Highlight text on a page.
    - Create your own figures, diagraming relations among concepts or timelines of events.
  ○ Involve the senses.
    - Give new dimensions to the words on the page. Smell the gunpowder of the revolutionary battle. Hear the chanting voices of thousands of protesters demanding their rights.
    - Imagine the person's name written in large, colorful letters.
    - If you compose a catchy jingle or rhyme, you'll remember that content for a very long time.
    - Construct mental images. Want to remember the town "Hopkinton"? Picture your cousin (your "kin") hopping onto a one-ton weight.
  ○ Make it important to you.
    - Trying to memorize the locations of historical events? Imagine yourself traveling to each location.
    - Imagine using the knowledge gained at a conference to solve a problem your company faces.
    - Think of the joy a friend will feel when you remember the dates of an upcoming vacation and follow up with her afterwards.
- Build a strong memory.
  ○ Memories tend to become less vivid over time, but you can build up a memory that will retain the important details. One way to retain those details is to study them multiple times, and in multiple ways.
    - When memorizing names before an event, you don't have to choose between writing the names out, thinking of associations you have with the names, or setting them to song. You can do all of these things! The more of them you do, the greater the likelihood that you will remember the names when the time comes.

- If you're trying to remember historical events, don't just look at them from one perspective; think about how each party would view the event.
- When learning a biochemical pathway, think what would happen if different parts of the system broke down because an enzyme was malfunctioning or the substrate was missing. Which substances would accumulate and which would run out?

9

Retrieve that memory

You studied hard. You drew out diagrams and created your own flash-cards. Yet, here you are, staring at a short-answer question on the exam and drawing a complete blank. You know you've generated this content from memory before, but you can't bring it to mind right now. You feel your heart racing faster as you try the next question, but it's the same problem—you're sure you know the answer, but you just can't think of it!

WHY DO THESE FAILURES OF MEMORY HAPPEN?

A lot has to go right for memory to succeed. You have to get the information *into* your memory and *keep* it there (as we covered in Chapter 8), and you also need to bring that information *back out* when relevant. Sometimes everything works seamlessly, and the content you need comes to mind easily. But, at other times, memory retrieval is more like bobbing for apples: The content you're searching for may be there, but no matter how hard you try, you cannot access it.

Retrieval failures are fairly common. At one time or another, we have all found ourselves searching for the name of an acquaintance or looking into our pantry trying to remember what we were going to get. Usually, this knowledge returns at a later moment—often when it is no longer of use to us. We think of the name once we're out of earshot or remember that we wanted to check whether we had enough pasta only after we begin preparing the sauce. Because the knowledge does eventually return to mind, we know the failure wasn't in getting information into memory, it was in getting the information back out. It was a failure of *retrieval* from memory.

CONSTRUCTING A MEMORY

Despite being so common, these memory retrieval failures often catch us off guard. In part, this may be because many of us rely on misleading metaphors to understand how memory works. If we think of memories as if they are books stored in a library or papers stored in a file cabinet, then retrieval failures should be relatively uncommon. But the truth is that there isn't "a memory" sitting somewhere in our brains waiting to be rediscovered. As we mentioned in the last chapter, a better metaphor for memory might be a structure built from blocks. The building blocks (brain cells and connections between them) are assembled as an event is experienced and stored as a memory. This memory "structure" does not, however, stay glued together in your brain. It is quickly disassembled so that other memories can be formed with those building blocks; only the "blueprints" (or *engram*[1]) of the memory remains. To retrieve the memory, it requires an *active process of reassembling* those blocks so that the memory can be rebuilt and the past experience can be accessed. If we use this metaphor, it can help us to understand many of the reasons why we can fail to retrieve information that we have initially stored.

INTERFERENCE

One frequent reason why retrieval fails is because you have some specific information "in mind" that makes it difficult to recall similar material. It's probably hard to recall what you ate for lunch two Thursdays ago, because your memory for all the lunches before and after it *interfere* with your ability to retrieve that specific lunch. You can think of it as having built a series of structures that are only subtly different from one another. Soon after building one of those memory structures, it's fairly easy to rebuild it: You can probably remember what you ate for lunch yesterday afternoon or, with effort, the day before that. But, over time, it becomes much more difficult—or even impossible—to rebuild one specific memory. Interference pushes you to build a prototypical "lunch memory," making it easier for you to recall where you *often* sit and who you *typically* eat with, while simultaneously making it harder to retrieve any *specific* memory of eating lunch. Having quick access to *typical* experiences is incredibly important for efficient decision-making—it's what allows you to generalize from one airport to another, or from one restaurant to another—but it can lead to frustrations when you don't want the details of a *typical* airport but instead to remember whether the terminal you are leaving from tomorrow has a restaurant where you can eat a sit-down meal before your flight.

Sometimes you may create your own interference through your efforts to come up with the right content, exacerbating your retrieval problems. As you see your acquaintance approach, you try to generate her name. You may feel that you're *nearly able* to retrieve the content—you may be certain that it's on the "tip of your tongue."[2] You think to yourself, "Is her name Sadie? Or Sarah?" These efforts, while well intentioned, can actually make it harder to retrieve the correct name (Sally). You have inadvertently *blocked* the desired content by bringing to mind similar, interfering content.

Interference can also arise from distractions in your environment. When you opened the pantry door to check how much pasta was on the shelf, you may have noticed that a box of cereal was left open. While you closed it—and wondered how many more times you would need to remind your daughter to close the box after breakfast—you forgot the task of checking for pasta. Only later, with another cue (like preparing the pasta sauce) do you remember.

STRESS

When you can't retrieve a memory in the desired moment, it can create *stress*. You might feel your palms becoming sweaty as you realize you can't recall the name of your acquaintance who is walking toward you. Unfortunately, stress makes retrieval failures even more likely to arise or to persist. As we discussed in Part 1, the *hippocampus,* deep in the temporal lobe, stores the blueprints and orchestrates the memory reassembly process. As it guides that reassembly process, the hippocampus also acts like tape, fastening multiple building blocks together to create a memory filled with content that you can consciously access. Stress can be disruptive to the functioning of the hippocampus, making it hard to efficiently rebuild the memory and retrieve the content you're looking for. Under stress, you might not find the blueprints to begin assembling the memory, or the first blocks you assemble might begin to detach as you attempt to insert additional blocks into your memory structure.

Now, you might be remembering back to Chapter 8 and thinking, "But wait: I thought emotions and stress could be helpful for getting information into my memory!" Indeed, the biochemical environment that is established when you're stressed seems to help you get at least some critical content *into* memory, but that same biochemical environment can actually prevent you from getting content *back out* of memory. When you're stressed, your brain prioritizes your ability to figure out what's going on in the environment *right now*. It deprioritizes those processes that would allow you to gain access to content from a *prior* moment in time—which is, of course, exactly what you need for memory retrieval to succeed.

This is a key reason why exam anxiety can be so disruptive to a student's ability to show what they have learned in a class. The stress will make it much harder for the student to retrieve the needed content from their days of studying. At the same time, that stress is likely to sear the exam-taking experience into the student's memory: "The teacher announced only 10 minutes remaining. There I sat, unable to figure out the right answer." This experience can, in turn, provoke anxiety as the next exam approaches, creating a vicious cycle of stress-induced poor memory retrieval.

NEVER THE SAME WAY

Let's turn to another key feature of memory: *You tend not to remember the same event in exactly the same way twice*. Each retrieval is slightly different, because each time you rebuild a memory, you approach its construction in a slightly different way.[3] Sometimes the differences are so subtle that they may be impossible to notice. At other times, they may give rise to a completely different interpretation of a past event or emphasize a very different part of the content.

Let's try an exercise for a minute. Think back to a special event that occurred when you were in high school. Perhaps it was a dance, an important game, an assembly, or graduation day. Spend a moment trying to bring all the features to mind.

You may have focused on any number of details: the clothes you were wearing or the way your surroundings looked, the people you were with or the topics of conversation, the emotions you were experiencing or the thoughts running through your mind. It is unlikely that any single retrieval would include *all possible* details; we rarely use each and every feature to rebuild the memory. Each time we rebuild the memory, we use a slightly different subset of features, and we create a new structure to represent the memory.[4] For these reasons, the details you focus on *now* may differ from the details you focused on at other times when you brought this memory to mind.

WHAT GUIDES HOW MEMORIES ARE REASSEMBLED?

Sometimes it's hard to pinpoint reasons for the differences between one retrieval and another. Why did Elizabeth remember picking out the dress she had worn under her polyester royal blue graduation gown today, when she hadn't thought of that detail in years? Other times, the reasons are more obvious. When Elizabeth described her high school graduation to her young daughter—who was about to participate in a preschool graduation ceremony—her memory focused primarily on logistics and feelings: Elizabeth shared with her daughter how she had walked from one end of the stage to the other and shook the hand of her principal while accepting her diploma, and how she had initially felt nervous on stage but then looked out at the audience and felt better when she saw her family and friends. When Elizabeth reminisced about that same graduation at a recent high school reunion, her memories centered on comedic moments, the teachers, and the physical campus—noting where they had their picture taken after graduation, and how there was a new building in the middle of the procession route. The *reason* the memory was being retrieved was different in these two cases, and so the details that sprang to mind also differed. These differences emphasize that memory retrieval isn't just something that happens spontaneously—it can also be a process you consciously or unconsciously guide, with your goals and motivations shaping how the retrieval unfolds.

USE THE RIGHT CUE

The reminiscences in the example above highlight how moments that are seemingly forgotten can return to mind with the right *retrieval cue*. Perhaps you experienced the effectiveness of a retrieval cue when we asked you to search for a memory from high school; you may have remembered an event that you hadn't reflected on for quite some time. *General cues* that anchor you to a past phase of your life (high school, for example) can be particularly useful for bringing to mind past events. These general cues give you *just enough* information to help you start rebuilding a memory.

Specific cues can be a double-edged sword. Sometimes they can help you to think of details you haven't recalled in some time. At her high school reunion, one of Elizabeth's classmates mentioned how they had to wait in the hot gym before the procession. As soon as it was mentioned, Elizabeth vividly remembered it: sitting on the bleachers, crowded together next to friends, their gowns sticking to them in the humidity, and their nervous chatter and disbelief that they were about to graduate. All it took was that simple cue reminding her of waiting in the gym for Elizabeth's graduation memory to be reassembled from details she had not thought of in some time.

But a word of warning: You need to be wary about whether any newly-added content retrieved from a specific cue is accurate. As we'll explore more in Chapter 12, we are all susceptible to incorporating *misinformation*—erroneous or misleading details—into our memories. We can all too easily incorporate someone else's embellishments into our own memories or distort or merge details from events based on someone else's suggestions. Was that memory of sitting on the gym bleachers really from graduation day? Or might it have been a memory from a final all-school assembly, when students were first handed their graduation gowns and—despite admonitions to wait until they were home—immediately ripped off the plastic wrapper and rushed to slip them on over their clothes right then and there?

Not only can specific cues from other people sometimes lead to memory distortions, they also can actually *hinder* your retrieval of other memory details. If you begin talking with a relative about the entrée at your cousin's wedding, this cue may make it relatively easy for you to remember the things that happened while you were seated for the dinner (because brain activity is increased for this part of the memory), but it may make it harder to remember the things that happened earlier at the cocktail hour or later on the dance floor (because brain activity is inhibited for these related but different parts of the memory, as if they were competing with each other for attention). By being reminded of one part of a memory, it's like you've shined a bright spotlight on a corner of a dimly lit room—although that corner is easy to see, the contrast makes the rest of the room harder to discern. Overall, you may end up recalling fewer details from the wedding than you otherwise would have because of the cue you were given.

CUES FOR THE FUTURE

Have you ever intended to stop at the grocery store on the way home, but then forgotten to do so as you drove past the turnoff? These *prospective memory*[5] errors arise when we make a plan for a future time, and then fail to execute that plan when the moment arises. These errors can be frustrating and, in the case of failing to remember to take medications, even dangerous.

In the absence of using external reminders, the best way to minimize these errors is to create strong retrieval cues, and to rehearse them repeatedly. Imagine yourself turning left onto the road that takes you to the grocery store; feel your hand on the turn signal, think of the landmarks at that turn. Bring that image to mind when you first realize you need to stop at the grocery store. Bring it to mind again as you walk toward your car after work. By making those strong associations, you're more likely to remember to execute your plan—to turn left and head toward the grocery store—when the moment arises.

CONTEXT MATTERS

How you retrieve a memory can be influenced not only by the cues given to you by others but also by the *context* in which you find yourself at that moment. At the broadest level, you can think of context as including both your inner state (the mood you're in, the reason you're retrieving a memory right now) and your external environment (your physical surroundings, the people you are with). Each of these can have a large impact on how you remember an event.

Examples abound in which your internal state influences the way you remember your past. If you are thinking about a romantic relationship because it has just ended, you are likely to bring to mind different details of past events than if you are focusing on the same relationship while happily celebrating an anniversary. If you are sad, you are more likely to remember sad events—past events that are consistent with that mood. If you are reminiscing with a friend in an effort to cheer them up, you are likely to focus on positive moments from your shared past. All these examples reflect ways in which your internal state will influence not only which memories you will recall but also how you reassemble those memories.

Your external environment also serves as a powerful retrieval cue. If you return to your childhood hometown, you are likely to think about events that you haven't thought about in some time. Seeing the corner store may remind you of saving your allowance to buy comic books. Passing the library may remind you of the story time hours and puppet shows that you cherished as a child but haven't thought about in years. The physical environment gives you a set of retrieval cues that can help bring past events to mind.

RETRIEVE THE WAY YOU LEARNED

These examples highlight a key principle of memory: Retrieval is most likely to succeed when you have access to the same information that was available to you when you first built the memory. In a famous experiment, participants studied material either on land or underwater—yes, you read that correctly— and were then tested in one of those two locations.[6] Participants who studied and were tested in the same location did better than those who had a location change in between study and test. Having the same context (such as location in this example) helps you to find the cues you need to reassemble the memory in a way that more closely approximates the memory's original construction. So does studying material in a similar way to how you will later be tested: Flashcards won't be of much use for an all-essay exam, and a focus on translating English into French would not serve you well if your teacher expects you to trans- late French into English.

SO MANY WAYS TO FAIL RETRIEVING THAT MEMORY

With the knowledge gained in this chapter, you are now ready to understand all the different reasons why you might have had trouble taking the exam in the example that we presented at the chapter's outset. You might have experienced interference from similar items—perhaps even from items you generated yourself trying to answer the questions. As you struggled, you experienced stress, which only made it more difficult to retrieve the right answers. The exam might have presented a cue that helped you retrieve some of the items more easily while actually blocking you from retrieving others. If you usually studied in your room in the late afternoon with a coffee at hand and you're taking the exam in the morning at a specialized testing center that doesn't allow food and drink, then there is a mismatch for both your internal and external context. Lastly, you may have studied the content in one way, but the exam was asking you for it in a different way. You may have studied using flashcards, which may not have been helpful on short-answer questions that required integration of multiple concepts.

HOW TO MINIMIZE RETRIEVAL FAILURES

Here are some key steps you can take when trying to remember information, such as someone's name or the correct answer on an exam.

- **Try to relax.**
  - This can be easier said than done, but relaxing can often be the most helpful antidote to retrieval failures because stress is so disruptive to retrieval. You may need to experiment with different ways to relax in these moments. Try taking a few slow, deep breaths as you feel your belly expand. Remind yourself that everyone has retrieval failures. Remember that the retrieval failure may just be temporary, and the information may return to mind shortly. If you find you can't diminish your stress, look for ways to take control of some aspects of it.
  - Still can't remember someone's name? Focus on being friendly instead, and the name may come once you're relaxed.
  - The first section of the exam looks impossible? Remember all the things you know and move on to a different section where you can feel more confident.
- **Minimize interference and blocking.**
  - Resist the urge to generate possible names for your acquaintance.
  - Don't try all possible completions to a fill-in-the-blank exam question.
- **Create general retrieval cues.**

- ○ Bring to mind a memory of your acquaintance (recall the last time you saw them or the person who introduced the two of you) or review other things you know about them, such as their work or family.
- ○ Outline the broad concepts related to the exam topic. Recalling this general information can set up additional context for the information you are seeking that can aid in your ability to bring the desired details to mind—without causing interference or blocking by mistake.
- **Try to return to the internal and external context of your learning, when possible.**
  - ○ Although you cannot teleport your acquaintance to where you first learned their name, you can still mentally time-travel and think about when you last saw them, picturing the location, ambiance, and other people present. You can also work to match your mood (happy, sad, concerned, silly) and the thoughts you were having at the time. These are all retrieval cues that will help to bring their name to mind.
  - ○ The same advice holds true for classroom exams. If you're having a retrieval failure, do what you can to get back into the context you were in while you studied. Picture yourself studying in your room: Imagine the layout of your textbook or your class notes. If you listened to music when you were studying, it may help to bring to mind one of the songs that played frequently during your study sessions.
  - ○ For classroom exams, it may also be tempting to modify your study context to match that in which you will need to retrieve the information, such as studying in the same classroom where you will be tested. But, as we briefly mentioned in Chapter 8, when preparing for an exam, you have the benefit (if you plan ahead and don't cram) of studying in multiple different contexts. Study in the library, in your room, and outdoors if the weather is nice. Review material in the morning and just before bed. Quiz yourself while drinking coffee and eating an apple—and also with no food or drink in sight. By doing so, you are broadening the set of contexts in which the information will be accessible. After all, you don't just want to remember your French vocabulary when

you are taking your midterm—you want to remember it when you are in Paris.

- **Try to acquire content in the same way that you will need to retrieve it.**
  - ○ There is nothing wrong with reviewing the names of the people you are likely to see at a social event later that day. To make such reviewing most helpful, look at their faces from photos or social media and then try to generate their names. For example, prior to attending a reunion, review yearbook photos and try to recall each name as you look at their faces.
  - ○ For exams, don't just study material the way it is presented in the textbook; think about how the teacher is most likely to test you and study the material that way. Not sure how you will be tested? Study the material multiple ways, so that however you will be tested, you will be ready.

10

Associate information

Across the room, a woman is smiling and waving at you. Her face is familiar. But how do you know her? She approaches and begins talking with you. It is only when she says how nice it was to meet you last weekend that you finally recall seeing her at your friend's birthday party. Suddenly, other details return: You remember she has a niece around your age and that you discussed your mutual enjoyment of hiking.

REMEMBERING THE DETAILS

Have you had an experience like this, when you recognize that you've seen someone or been somewhere before, but you cannot bring to mind any other details? Most people have these experiences from time to time. These moments typically arise because information, like a person's face or a stretch of road, can elicit a sense of *familiarity*—the recognition that a person or place is familiar—even when the information is insufficient to prompt you to remember other details.[1] Let's explore why this happens.

PUTTING IT TOGETHER

Remembering details—a process referred to as *recollection*—requires you to connect different pieces of information together. In previous chapters, we've analogized memory as the process by which structures are built and later reassembled. The prefrontal cortex—the part of the brain behind your forehead—helps you to select the details that ought to be included in the structure. The hippocampus—that seahorse-shaped structure deep within our brain—and the tissue surrounding it are essential for connecting that content, acting as the fastener that connects different building blocks together, ensuring that your memory structure is neither a series of disconnected rooms nor simply a bare scaffolding. These regions work together to build a memory structure that constitutes a prior event of your life (see Figure 10.1).

Creating a memory structure with connected details can be a relatively easy task if you already have some previous knowledge that helps you to link the details together. Remembering that your nephew loves marshmallows in his hot chocolate may be fairly easy to learn if you have prior knowledge that many children enjoy this combination. Remembering that he has a stuffed dragon named Rocket may be a harder association to retain; to do so, you might need to think about the fact that dragons and rockets both fly, or create a mental image of your nephew and a dragon going up into space on a rocket. In other words, holding on to these more arbitrary associations in memory requires effort, and can be helped by many of the same strategies to create a durable memory that we described in Chapter 8.

When memory structures get built (encoded) and stuck together (stored) with their rooms (the details) all interconnected, at retrieval you can often use memory for one detail to help you retrieve other, associated details. In the example at the beginning of this chapter, once memory for the birthday party

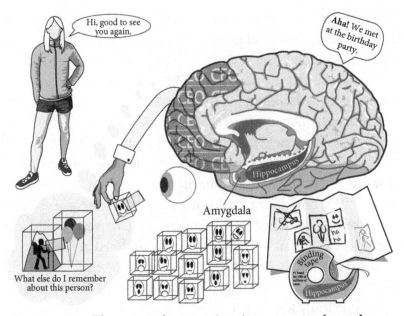

Figure 10.1. The central executive in your prefrontal cortex ("CEO" pattern, near your eye) and the hippocampus in your temporal lobe facilitate the recollection of detailed sights, sounds, and thoughts that together constitute an event of your life. The amygdala helps process the emotions of your recollected memory.

returned to your mind, so did your memory for other details about your prior encounter with the woman. It's as if standing in one room of your memory structure can reveal the corridor that can lead you into another room with another set of details.

But sometimes the prefrontal cortex or hippocampus fails to do its job. Often, the failure is at retrieval: The rooms and corridors exist, but the prefrontal cortex and hippocampus don't work together to allow the hippocampal index (described in Chapter 4) to reveal them. It's as if you're looking at the memory structure from a distance: You have only a vague feeling of familiarity, without any details. These failures are often transient, as in the example at the start of the chapter. Eventually, with the right retrieval cue, you're suddenly able to step into the relevant memory structure, moving beyond this feeling of familiarity as you recall more and more of the details.

At other times, the prefrontal cortex or hippocampus fails to do its job in the earlier stages of memory creation or storage. Perhaps the scaffolding for the memory structure is built but the rooms are not constructed. Or maybe the rooms are crafted but never adequately linked together. In these cases, you can still recognize that you've seen someone or something before—you have that feeling of familiarity—but you can't retrieve the details. You might wander down a street, realizing you've been there before, but unable to remember when. Or you might have a conversation that begins like the one outlined at the start of this chapter but ends with you still unable to recall the details of your past encounter—and without any details about this person who clearly knows you.

TYPES OF ASSOCIATIONS

There are many different types of information that you may want to build into your memory structure. They are similar in that they require the prefrontal cortex to select those details as important to be included in the memory structure and the hippocampus to serve as the Velcro—keeping those details bound within the structure. But each type of detail requires slightly different strategies for getting it into or out of your memory.

Name That Source

You often need to create a link between a piece of information and the context in which you encountered it. Did you learn something from a news outlet you trust, or was it from a social media post? Which parent told you about their child's trip to the emergency room due to a nut allergy? These details can be critical for good decision-making: Should you repeat the story to a colleague? Can you serve Nutella at tonight's event?

Despite their importance, these source details often don't get built into memory structures.[2] Attention to other details is often the cause. As you were reading the story, you might not have given much thought to its source, and so that detail may never have been committed to memory. As you were listening to the parent talk about their child, you may have been focused on the harrowing details of the event, rather than on who was telling the story. Building the source into your memory structure often takes extra effort. You can't take it for granted that you will be able to remember who said what, when, and where. If those details matter, you need to attend to them and take extra effort to commit them to memory.

Even if the source details do get incorporated into your memory structure, it takes additional effort at retrieval to bring them to mind again. So, if you're rushed or stressed—factors that tend to push you toward faster, less effortful ways to retrieve information from memory—you're more likely to just repeat the story you read, without considering whether it was from a trustworthy source. When the stakes are high (as in the nut allergy example), it can be important to slow down and give yourself a moment to check your mental sources before using or sharing the content you have stored in memory.

Who Did I Tell?

A related type of association is not who told you something, but to whom you told something. Have you ever launched into a story and—when you're halfway through—wondered if this is the second time you're telling it to this friend? Errors in *destination memory*[3] can become exacerbated as adults grow older, and they become even more pronounced with Alzheimer's disease or other forms of dementia (see Chapter 13). But all of us can suffer from these lapses. As with source memory errors, often the lapses result from inattention to the destination details: You may have been so caught up in relaying the story in just the right way that you didn't really focus on your audience. Other times, the problem is that you fail to monitor your memory for those details: Had you taken an extra moment to think back to when you'd previously told the story, you would have remembered telling it to this friend. But the story fit so well with the topic of conversation that, instead, you quickly jumped into its (re)telling.

Actions Versus Imaginations

You are driving to the airport and suddenly think: "Did I pack my passport—or did I only think about doing it?" Despite how important it is to determine whether you performed an action or only imagined it, it is often difficult to distinguish between these possibilities. There is tremendous overlap between how you use your brain to *imagine* an action and how you use your brain to actually *perform* that action. It takes about the same amount of time to imagine an action as to actually perform it, and similar brain networks are recruited whether you imagine or execute the action. This is one reason why, as described in Chapter 2, imagining motor actions can help us to improve at those skills. This similarity also means a memory for an imagined action will have a similar structure to a memory for a performed action—which can make them hard to distinguish from one another.

You can make the distinction a bit easier if, as you perform an action, you pay attention to features that you would be unlikely to imagine. As you pack your passport, you can pay attention to the texture of the passport cover, compare its size to the palm of your hand, and attend to how it looks placed in its safe location in your bag. You can also make it less likely that you will confuse your imaginings with reality if you build into your imagery some details that disconnect it from the present moment. For example, if you are imagining packing your passport as a way to help you remember to do so later, you might imagine yourself wearing a different outfit than the one you're currently wearing or think about the importance of performing the action at a later time of day, when the sun is setting.

Ordering Events

What about if you need to associate events on a timeline or in chronological order, such as a sequence of historical events or your recent trip itinerary?

In some cases (such as the sequence of historical events), you may be able to build one memory structure that would contain all of those temporal relations. Many mnemonics are designed to help retrieve content in a particular order every time. For instance, the "peg word" technique is a mnemonic that has you first memorize 10 items in order (1 = gun, 2 = shoe, 3 = tree, etc.) and then imagine the content you want to remember as being associated with those words. For instance, if trying to memorize the order of certain battles in the Civil War, you might imagine the *guns* in use first at Fort Sumner, then associate *shoe* with the Battle of Bull Run, *tree* with the Battle of Seven Pines, and so forth (see Chapter 25 for discussion of mnemonic devices).

In other cases (such as recalling the order in which you saw various sights on a recent trip), the desired information is likely to be spread across multiple different memory structures that were built throughout your trip. Sometimes, the information contained within one of these memories contains clues to order. You may remember wearing a necklace to the theater, and if you also know you bought that necklace in a museum store on that same trip, you can determine that you visited the museum before the theater. Other times, to figure out the order, you need to compare across different memory structures, which can be quite challenging. Recent evidence suggests that one of the reasons you can sometimes figure out these timing comparisons is because cells in some portions of the hippocampus show gradual time-dependent changes in the ways that they respond.[4] This means that a memory structure built on Day 1 of your trip will have a slightly different time signature than a memory structure built on Day 2, providing a kind of time-stamp to our memories. But gaining conscious access to those time signatures appears to be difficult, and time perception errors in memory abound.

Once More, with Feeling

Sometimes, what you want to remember is the emotion associated with an event. How did you feel on your graduation day? The emotions tied to an event are thought to exist in the amygdala (an almond-shaped structure just in front of the hippocampus) or in connections between the hippocampus and the amygdala. But, unlike other types of details that we've described, these features are subjective, and thus the emotions that you conjure when recalling a memory can have as much to do with your current emotional state as with the one you were in at the time the event occurred. If you have felt better about an event after talking about it with a friend, you recognize that the emotions tied to memories are malleable. Fortunately, over time, negative emotions are particularly likely to fade,[5] perhaps related to sleep (see Chapter 20). You might know that you were seething with anger during an argument but, years later, it is unlikely that you will fully re-experience that anger when reflecting back on the exchange.

The elicitation of strong emotions during an event can also affect the likelihood that other event details are remembered. There is still much ongoing work on this topic, but there is reason to think that negative emotions tend to "telescope" memories, giving good resolution to details linked to the negative experience (you might remember your friend's tone of voice or the look on her face during the argument) at the expense of other details (you may have no idea where the argument took place or who else was in the room).[6] Positive emotions may instead broaden the scope of the memory, making it easier to link together otherwise unrelated event elements.

THE IMPORTANCE OF KEEPING IT TOGETHER

Retaining the details of past events can be essential for good decision-making. The examples we've described highlight that it's often insufficient to have a single piece of information in mind to make the right decision. You also need to evaluate whether you should trust that piece of information, share it with someone, or follow through on an intention. In addition, there are other times when additional details serve as important building blocks for other key functions of memory.

Building Inferences

Inferences allow you to build upon your prior knowledge to make sense of the present moment. The root of inferential learning is your ability to form associations in memory—and then to pull those associations back out of your memory when needed. This ability can be a key to learning in classroom settings as well as in daily life.

If you see a child being picked up at daycare by a man one day and by a woman the next day, you probably wouldn't be surprised to later see the man and woman together. You would have effortlessly made the inference that they know one another, through their shared association with the child,[7] without needing to see them together. But that inference—that new association between the man and the woman—can only be made if, upon seeing the child with the woman, you remember previously seeing the child with the man.

Similarly, if you see a woman holding a diaper, you can use your preexisting knowledge to infer that there is a baby nearby, even if you never see that baby. But again, that inference can only be made if you've built a strong association between diapers and babies; if that association isn't brought to mind, then the inference can't be made.

Update That Memory

Associating details together also helps to keep our memories up to date. Your friend may have pursued a PhD in biology, but later decided to change career paths to become a photographer. Another friend may have married, taking her spouse's last name. In both cases, you must update your knowledge about your friend, creating a new association. Equally importantly, you want those new associations to be the ones that come to mind—rather than the older ones—so that you don't continue to ask your one friend about her latest biology experiment or refer to your other friend by her maiden name. Fortunately, the time signatures in the hippocampus that we described earlier can help with this: The memory structures that have a time signature closer to the present moment will generally come to mind first, allowing you to remember which is your friend's current career or last name.

HOW TO KEEP IT TOGETHER

Now that you know how important it can be to remember the details, here's what you can do to more effectively build those details into your memory structure and access them when needed.

- **Attend to the details you want to remember.** Does this advice sound familiar? We keep repeating it because it is so important. If you don't want to forget where you read a story, be sure to attend to your sources. Pay attention to the title of a book or to the outlet you're reading online. If you don't want to tell the same story to the same person twice, pay close attention to who is with you as you tell the story; closely considering their facial expressions and reactions to the story will help. If you're at a specific event (perhaps a wedding or a reunion), make a mental note of the occasion on which you've told the story.

- **Link the details together.** It's hard to create a mental structure that consists of unrelated content, so put in the effort to connect the details. Build those corridors that can connect one room of your structure to the next. Both the corridors and the effort of building them will help.
  - *Do this verbally*: It can be something as simple as saying aloud, "I'm putting my keys on the dresser," or repeating the phrase, "key–dresser." Or try creating a novel statement like, "My dresser holds the key."
  - *Use mental imagery*: Imagine standing on top of a mountain with the new acquaintance with whom you're discussing your enjoyment of hiking.
  - *Use mnemonic devices*: If you find yourself often needing to remember associations or long lists of information, you may benefit from taking the time to train yourself in the use of mnemonic devices. See Chapter 25.
- **Try different retrieval cues.** As you try to find your keys, imagine yourself coming home earlier or actually retrace your footsteps as you walked in the door. If you're trying to remember who told you about their child's nut allergy, bring to mind any details you do remember: Where did you have the conversation? What else did you talk about with this parent?
- **Stay calm.** We've said this before, but it bears repeating: Stress is particularly harmful for constructing—and reconstructing—memory structures that contain all the relevant details. We fully recognize it can be difficult to stay calm as you're rushing to find your misplaced keys or feeling uneasy when you can't recall where you met someone. But take a deep breath, remember that memory lapses like these are common and often transient, and focus on what you can do in the moment—like trying those different retrieval cues.

11

Control what you forget and remember

It's your first day at a new job, and as you walk into a conference room, you trip over a power cable and nearly fall. You feel yourself blush and hope that not too many people saw the stumble. The next day, as you walk into the conference room, you think of this unpleasant moment. This is one memory you'd like to forget. If only there were a way to stop unwanted memories from coming to mind!

Would you like to be able to control what you remember *and* what you forget?

You may often think about forgetting as a consequence of having an imperfect memory system. But sometimes, as in the example above, you may be particularly motivated to forget information: You may not want an unpleasant event to spring to mind at inopportune moments, or you may recognize that information is unimportant and not worth remembering. In this chapter, we'll explore the extent to which you can control what you remember—and what you forget.

CONTROLLING WHAT DETAILS GO INTO MEMORY

As a college professor, Elizabeth knows that few things can get students to pay attention like saying, "This is going to be on the exam." Although you can be imperfect in implementing your plans, you know that when something is important to remember, you should pay attention. More generally, when you know there is value to information—that it will help you on a later exam or job interview—your brain prioritizes getting that information into your memory. There are specialized neural circuits that are engaged by reward that can enhance your ability to get information into memory, making it more likely that the hippocampus does a good job and builds a memory structure replete with details.

Tag It in the Past

You can even learn *after an event is over* that its details were important, and that knowledge can increase the likelihood those details will be sustained over time in the memory structure you built.[1] Imagine leaving your eighth-floor office and walking home, only to find upon arriving at your front door that you've lost your keys. Suddenly, details of your chosen path that may have seemed irrelevant at the time—which elevator you rode down to the lobby, which side of the road you walked along—take on a new importance. At least for a while after an event has occurred, you can *reprioritize* event details, bringing to the forefront details that you suddenly realize have high importance.

Forget That Memory

The converse is also true: If you tell someone that content is *unimportant* to remember, they won't do very well at retaining the information, even if they didn't realize its irrelevance when they first encountered it. For example, Robert Bjork at the University of California at Los Angeles showed participants lists of words and told them they would be tested on them later. But after one of the lists, participants were told that they were accidentally shown the wrong list, and those specific words wouldn't be tested. In reality, the participants' memories were tested for all of the words. The key result is that participants did worse at recalling the words from the list they were told they didn't need to remember.[2] It's as if, upon finding out that the information is not relevant, you can wipe your mental slate clean.

This ability to keep unwanted details out of your memory structures can be quite important, because sometimes it's not just that the information is irrelevant, but that the information is incorrect. If someone gives you erroneous information, it behooves you to wipe that detail from your memory structures and, if possible, to replace it with the correct content. Although none of us are perfect at doing this, when an error is identified soon after learning, these "intentional forgetting" mechanisms can reduce the likelihood that the error gets represented in your memory structure, minimizing your reliance on the faulty information for decision-making.[3]

These results emphasize that you can exert some control over the information that gets prioritized for building into your memory structures. Details can be removed from the construction when you realize they are unimportant or erroneous, and they can be added in high relief when their importance becomes apparent soon after learning.

CONTROLLING WHAT DETAILS YOU STORE INTERNALLY

Whether you realize it or not, you are constantly making choices that affect whether you store content internally in your brain or externally in the world. Do you attempt to memorize a shopping list or write it down with no expectation that you will remember the items without consulting the list? Do you try to learn the information you look up online or in a book, or only learn where to find it again the next time you need it?

You also may rely on the fact that other people can serve as your external memory aids.[4] You might rely on your business partner to remember clients' names, your spouse to keep track of where the recipe for a favorite dish is kept, and your child to recall the dates of their performances you plan to attend.

It can be quite helpful to "outsource" your memories in this way, and we'll talk about memory aids that help you to do this in Chapter 22. For example, it may not be worth the effort to memorize a list of grocery items, and it often isn't efficient for there to be high redundancy in the information that different members of a company—or a household—represent in memory. Indeed, higher rates of *transactional memory*—that tendency to rely on others' memories to supplement your own—tend to be related to better performance in businesses.[5] So, outsourcing memory can be a smart strategy in many circumstances. However, problems arise if you don't think through the repercussions of this offloading: If your business partner departs, is critical knowledge forever lost? If an oft-visited website is down for maintenance, what impact does this have on your ability to complete your task?

CONTROLLING WHICH DETAILS YOU ACCESS FROM MEMORY

So far in this chapter, we've focused on controlling what content *goes into* memory. The example we began the chapter with is instead an example of controlling the content we *pull back out of* our memory stores. It's also taken from a real event: During one of the first lectures that Elizabeth gave as a newly-minted professor, she tripped over a power cable and nearly fell fully onto the floor before she caught herself. The next class, as soon as she approached the location, that memory returned. The power cable was no longer there, and so it was not a helpful memory to have in mind while trying to remain composed at the front of the room. When the same memory sprang to mind the next class as well, Elizabeth set out to do something about it. When something cued her to think of that stumble— she walked past the part of the room where she had tripped, or saw a cable lying in another part of the room—she immediately tried to put the memory out of her mind. If she felt glimmers of the memory returning, she did all she could to squelch them, slamming on the mental brakes so that the full details of the event did not return to mind. It took a few classes, but soon the memory didn't spring to mind every time she walked around the classroom. Now, although Elizabeth regularly teaches in that room, she rarely thinks about that event.

These additional details about the event emphasize two important principles of how you can control what you access from memory. First, it's an *effortful* process. Elizabeth had to work to put the memory out of mind. Without putting in that effort, the memory probably would have continued to return for quite some time, cued by features in the room or by associations in Elizabeth's own mind. Second, it's not the same as erasing the memory. Elizabeth didn't give herself amnesia for the event; she can still recall the memory, but she reduced the likelihood that it would be one of the first memories to come to mind when she enters that room.

CONTROLLING THE EMOTION IN MEMORIES

Sometimes, you want to recall the content from a prior event, but you don't want to fully re-experience its emotions. It might be motivating for you to remember the time you didn't study enough for a final exam and wound up with a poor grade—you might be able to use that memory to help you hunker down and study for an upcoming test rather than socializing with friends. But it won't help you to be consumed with the negative emotions you experienced upon first receiving your grade.

Similar to how you control the details you access from memory, you can work to control the emotions within a memory. Sometimes, you can control the emotion elicited by a memory in parallel with your control of access to the memory content, suppressing access to both the content of a memory and its emotion.[6] Other times, you may be able to strategically regulate your emotions during memory retrieval so as to, over time, specifically dull the emotional facets of a memory while preserving other details in high relief.

PUTTING MEMORY CONTROL TO WORK

To best control what you remember and what you forget, try the following:

- **Create priority cues.** Think directly about why something is important (or unimportant) to remember. If you're listening to a professor, think to yourself, "This is likely to be on the exam." If you're listening to a friend talk about an upcoming trip, think, "I want to remember this so I can ask her about it later."
- **Be deliberate about outsourcing memory.** In this digital age, it's especially easy to rely on external memory aids, often without realizing you're doing it, such as how passwords auto-complete, social media sends birthday reminders, and phone numbers are stored in your phone. Give thought to what information you choose to store externally versus internally, so you can make sure the information you store in your brain is the information most useful to keep there!
- **Push it out of mind.** If you have an experience like Elizabeth, finding that an unwanted memory is coming to mind, research

from Michael Anderson and colleagues has shown that an effective strategy is to slam on your mental brakes, clearing your mind of the memory and forcing it from your consciousness.[7] It's important that you don't just distract yourself. Instead, work to actively snuff out the memory, just as you'd use a snuffer to extinguish a flame.

12

Are you sure that's not a false memory?

You are gathered around the dinner table with extended family, reminiscing about a prior Thanksgiving meal. The turkey wasn't ready to eat until at least 8 p.m. Everyone was so hungry! It was past your daughter's bedtime by the time the food was on the table, and she nearly fell asleep in her mashed potatoes. Everyone is laughing at the memory. But then your spouse gently interjects: Wasn't that dinner before our daughter was born? He remembers cousin Suzy being at that dinner but, in recent years, she's been spending Thanksgiving with her in-laws. You definitely remember your daughter being exhausted at that meal. But maybe Suzy was there . . . in which case it must have been before your daughter was born.

You've probably had a few moments like this one, when you transition from feeling confident in your memory to questioning some parts of it—maybe eventually realizing that an event could not have happened the way you remembered it.

Recall some of the reasons why memory errors occur, as we discussed in Chapters 7 through 9. You can't attend to everything, and so some details never make it into your memory structure. And, without meaning to, each time you retrieve a memory, you may subtly—or even not so subtly—change how you reconstruct its features, omitting some details and distorting others. Usually, those omissions or distortions are innocuous, but sometimes they can lead you to have a misleading impression of what happened. Even when you can definitively determine what happened—perhaps there was a social media post or diary entry about the event—you may never quite feel satisfied, because there is still an alternate version of the past floating around in your memory that feels real to you.

CONFIDENT, YET WRONG

Are memories usually correct if you are confident about them? Yes and no. In many circumstances, confidence is an imperfect yet reasonably good marker of memory accuracy; most research shows a positive association between the two.[1] But there can be important disconnects between the two, especially when information has been retrieved on multiple occasions or retold multiple times. In one clever experiment, researchers from Victoria University of Wellington in New Zealand and University of Victoria in British Colombia showed participants actual photos from their childhood intermixed with a photograph that was altered to create the appearance that the participant had been in a hot air balloon as a child.[2] The participants were interviewed three times over 1 to 2 weeks, and each time they were shown each photo and asked to remember everything they could about the event. As you might expect, no participant immediately reported a memory upon seeing the fake photograph; but by the end of the third interview, half of the participants reported at least some details of a hot air balloon ride. Moreover, when asked to rate their confidence in the false memory, they put themselves around the midpoint of the confidence scale.

Imagination Inflation

Why do false memories like this happen? A likely contributor
is that when you try to remember an event, you often imagine
what might have happened. If someone says you've eaten at a
restaurant before (but you have no memory of it) you're likely
to think about when you might have gone there, who you could
have eaten with, and what you may have ordered. Now you've
created a mental image, and once this mental image has been
created, it can be hard for you to figure out if it's *just* an imagining or if it's an actual memory. As we described in Chapter 10,
the construction of mental imagery relies on many of the same
processes required for action or perception. So, it's no wonder
that, after imagining how something might have occurred a
couple of times, you may come to believe that it really happened
that way.

Confidence-Boosting Feedback

Sometimes, you aren't confident in the content you've retrieved
from memory. You may guess an answer when called upon by
a teacher, or when asked yet another "why" question by your
grandchild. But if you receive feedback that you are probably
right—the professor responds, "good answer," or your grandchild says, "oh, right, my teacher said that"—you will suddenly
become much more confident in your answer. What's particularly interesting is that you don't just become more confident *now*; you also will remember being more confident *at the
time when you first responded*. You might not remember your
response was a guess; your memory may quickly convince you
that you confidently knew the answer all along.

This is one of the reasons why, in police and legal work, there
has been a push toward recording eyewitnesses' first identifications of a suspect. The confidence in that first moment of identification can be recorded and later considered by judge and
jury. The confidence of that first identification is a reasonably

good predictor of accuracy, and certainly a much better predictor than later estimates of confidence that may be affected by feedback or coaching. Importantly, confirming feedback can not only inflate confidence in an identification but also lead an eyewitness to believe they had a better view of the event or suspect than they actually had—influencing multiple factors that a judge and jury consider when trying to determine the reliability of eyewitness testimony.[3]

Distorting Sources and Blending Memories

It's often the case that our false memories aren't *entirely* false. They might have some elements of true memories blended together in a way that creates an erroneous impression of the past. In the example at the start of the chapter, perhaps there *was* a late-night Thanksgiving meal before your daughter was born *and also* a Thanksgiving dinner, years later, that overlapped with your daughter's afternoon naptime such that she'd been nearly asleep at the table. Over time, the memories may have become merged, preserving some details from each. The memories of the hot air balloon ride may similarly have contained elements from real events—perhaps of being high above the ground on a ride at a fairground, or of seeing a brightly-colored balloon and imagining the thrill of being in the air. These snippets—pulled out of actual memory structures and merged into one another—can set the foundation for a false memory.

The Power of Misinformation

You already know from earlier chapters that our memory for an event can easily be altered as we reconstruct the event's details at each retrieval. That alteration is very likely to occur when someone we trust suggests that an event unfolded in a particular way. When the suggestion is wrong, the phenomenon is referred to as the *misinformation effect*.[4] In one famous experiment by Elizabeth Loftus and colleagues,[5] participants saw a simulated car accident that included a car going through a *stop* sign. In later questioning about the accident, some participants were asked about the circumstances in which the car went through a *yield* sign. Many of those who received this misleading question came to remember that the original video had contained a yield sign rather than a stop sign. This same research team revealed that even subtle suggestions can influence memory. Participants who were asked how fast a car was going when it "bumped" into another car remembered lower speeds than those asked how fast it was going when it "crashed." So, perhaps cousin Suzy wasn't at that Thanksgiving dinner—but the confident assertion that she was there could lead to her incorporation into your memory.

Perhaps counterintuitively, *you* can be a powerful source of your own misinformation. One example is if you lie. Individuals who lie, saying that erroneous details occurred during an event, can come to believe that those details really happened. Similarly, individuals who speak about an event and then later deny that they spoke about it can forget that they actually discussed the event's details.[6] But even if you aren't attempting to deceive anyone, the way you reflect on past events—perhaps imagining some alternate versions ("what if . . .")—also has the potential to introduce misinformation.

SO MANY WAYS FOR MEMORY TO BECOME DISTORTED

In case you—or someone you're talking with about this book— need further convincing that false memories commonly arise, we're going to ask you to participate in a brief experiment, adapted from "the DRM paradigm," named for the three scientists who developed it: James Deese at Johns Hopkins University and Henry Roediger and Kathleen McDermott, both at Washington University in St. Louis.[7] Read the set of words after the bullet and, in a little while, we'll ask you to recall the ones that you remember:

• *Table, sit, legs, seat, couch, desk, recliner, sofa, cushion, stool, bed, rest, dream, awake, pillow, snore, slumber, candy, sour, bitter, sugar, cake, eat, tooth, pie*

You have a few advantages going into this task: You're reading a book that has already given you some tips on how to remember information, and you know that you're about to be quizzed on your memory. Even so, we anticipate that you may have a false memory. If not, you can try this experiment on a few friends; we anticipate that a least a few of them will.

Now, time for that memory test: Without looking back, what were those words on the list we presented earlier? There were a total of 25 words; take a minute or two to recall as many as you can.

If you're like most people, you'll do well remembering words toward the start of the list: *table, sit, legs.* This is called the primacy effect in memory, and it can also be seen for more complex events from our lives: It's much easier to remember your "firsts," whether it's your first kiss, first day of college, or first overseas flight, than it is to remember later repetitions of similar events. What about the other words on the list: Did you remember *sofa? bed? dream? candy? sugar?* What about *chair? sleep? sweet?* If you remembered any of those last three words, then you've just had a false memory! You can go back and check the list to confirm; none of those words were on it. We do these types of demonstrations for high school and college students, lawyers and judges, doctors and nurses, and it's always the same: A large proportion of people generate these non-presented words. Many are quite confident they were on the list. If you were someone who hadn't seen the original list of words and were just going by the show of hands in the room, you'd probably be fairly convinced that those words were on the list. In fact, more people recall those words than some of the actually-presented words!

If you reread the words that were presented, you can probably guess as to why this experiment leads to memory errors. The words you read were all closely associated with those non-presented words. In fact, the words you read were chosen specifically because they are strongly associated with the non-presented words. They represent the gist or general theme of the list. The words *chair, sleep,* or *sweet* might have even sprung to mind as you were reading the list of words—which would also cause these non-presented words to feel highly familiar to you if they came to mind when you were recalling the list. Moreover, when we asked you for the words, we tried to push you toward recalling as many of them as possible. We told you there were 25 words on the list because we know that most people won't be able to remember all 25 words, and knowing that you're "coming up short" can push you to accept as a memory whatever content springs to mind. This tendency is one reason why it is important that eyewitnesses are reminded that the perpetrator may not be in the lineup.

INFERRING TRUTH FROM FAMILIARITY

Answer quickly: What does a cow drink? The answer is of course water, but if your first thought was "milk," you aren't alone. Because milk is a beverage that we associate with cows, it will spring to mind quickly for many of us. Elizabeth does this demonstration aloud in class, asking students to shout out the answer as fast as they can: The first shouts are almost always "milk," and only a little later is "water" heard. When you're trying to respond quickly, it's easy to assume that the information that pops easily into your mind is accurate.

Another example of this tendency to accept information that pops into your head as accurate is the *illusory truth effect.*

This phenomenon describes the tendency to trust information that you've heard multiple times. This inclination to believe repeated information can be important for your ability to learn—a teacher might misspeak once, but they probably won't consistently generate wrong information—and children learn the association between repetition and truth by the time they are school-aged. But where this tendency pivots from being beneficial to damaging is that it continues to operate *even if you've been warned that the information is coming from an unreliable source* and *even if you've been directly told the information is false.* This phenomenon can be exploited by everyone from advertisers to politicians. It is particularly problematic on social media, a mode of communication that encourages superficial thinking (as you scan from one posting to another) and motivates the repetition and sharing of content.

With his colleagues Jason Mitchell and Dan Schacter, Andrew examined this illusory truth effect in older adults and individuals with Alzheimer's disease.[8] The participants in this experiment studied 44 ambiguous statements that were randomly assigned "true" or "false" labels, such as, "It takes 32 coffee beans to make a cup of espresso: FALSE," and "It takes 4 hours to hard boil an ostrich egg: TRUE." When participants were then asked which statements were true, healthy older adults correctly identified 77% of the true statements as being true, but they also identified 39% of the false statements as being true. Although this result is startling in itself, the Alzheimer's results are even more so. Individuals with Alzheimer's disease correctly identified 69% of the true statements as being true, but also identified 59% of the false statements as being true—more than the half you'd expect them to identify if they were just guessing. This means that if you tell an individual with Alzheimer's that some information isn't true, they may be more likely to remember that the information *is* true than if you didn't say anything at all. The bottom line is that you should never tell an individual with Alzheimer's what isn't true ("Don't take your medicine after dinner")—just tell them what is true ("Take your medicine on an empty stomach").

WHAT ABOUT THE ACCURACY OF EMOTIONAL MEMORIES?

At this point in the chapter, you may be thinking, "Well, sure, memories aren't always perfect, but there are some events that are forever etched in my memory, and I *know* that they are accurate." Perhaps it's your first kiss, the moment you first held your child in your arms, where you were when you first learned that John F. Kennedy was assassinated, who you were with when you saw the towers fall in the September 11, 2001, attacks, or what you were doing when you heard the 2016 election results. Many people are confident in their memory for these types of events—even when they happened decades ago—and you may feel like you are re-experiencing those moments as you recall them. The term "flashbulb memory" was coined in 1977 by two memory researchers from Harvard, Roger Brown and James Kulik, to describe the vivid way in which highly surprising, emotional, and important events seem to sear themselves into our memories—as if a flash photograph were taken, forever imprinting details of the event.

Picture-Perfect?

It turns out that emotional memories are not picture-perfect; they're actually prone to all the same types of distortions as other memories. Even Brown and Kulik recognized that it was not appropriate to consider emotional memories as like photographs in all respects, stating, "An actual photograph, taken by flashbulb, preserves everything within its scope; it is altogether indiscriminate. Our flashbulb memories are not." They go on to describe how, although they have vivid memories of where they were when they learned of the assassination of JFK, details are missing. For instance, they note that Brown "faced a desk with many objects on it, and some kind of weather was visible through the window, but none of this is in his memory picture."[9]

Confidence, Not Consistency

Although there can be some situations when emotional memories are remembered with better detail than more mundane experiences, what is most remarkable about memories for situations that evoke emotion is how vivid those memories feel to us and how confident we are about their accuracy—even when we're wrong. In one of the first demonstrations of this disconnect between confidence and accuracy for an emotional event, Ulrich Neisser and Nicole Harsh at Emory University asked college students to report the circumstances in which they learned about the explosion of the space shuttle Challenger.[10] Months later, they were asked to again report those circumstances and to rate their confidence in their memory. Participants gave detailed reports at both timepoints, and were highly confident in their memory's accuracy, yet many details were inconsistent. This disconnect between confidence and accuracy (or, at least, consistency) in emotional memories has since been demonstrated for many different public events, leading Jennifer Talarico and David Rubin at Duke University to publish a paper with the title "Confidence, Not Consistency, Characterizes Flashbulb Memories."[11]

Rehearsal Boosts Confidence

As noted by Ken Paller at Northwestern University, one reason for this disconnect between confidence and accuracy may relate to how frequently we think about past emotional experiences.[12] We reflect on these events and discuss them with others. Each time, we build a memory structure for the event. After so much rehearsal, the construction process begins to feel effortless, and the structure created seems like a replica of the original event. But in reality, each of those rebuildings provides an opportunity for us to misplace or omit a block, to incorporate erroneous content from someone else's comments, or to morph our structure based on knowledge we learned after the fact.

Remembering the Threat

Another reason for this disconnect between confidence and accuracy may be that there is some, relatively small, subset of details that we may remember extremely well from an emotional event. The *weapon focus effect* describes how individuals have more trouble identifying a suspect, and have more false identifications, if a weapon is visible.[13] This isn't simply because people don't see the other details.[14] It's as if all the brain's resources are being devoted toward building that threat (whether a gun, knife, or menacing fist) into the memory structure and other details (like the perpetrator's face or clothing) are inadequately constructed. Later, if we are asked to think about the event as a whole, we may feel like we have a vivid memory because of the select portions that are so crisply retained. It's as if we're standing in one room of our memory structure, marveling at the gilded relief in which some details are portrayed, without realizing that the corridors that should have led to other details have crumbled.

PROTECTING AGAINST FALSE MEMORIES

What can you do to defend yourself against false memories? The most important piece of advice is: If the stakes are high, take the time to monitor your memory. After content has come to mind, consider *why* that content might have come to mind, and evaluate whether it is the right content. Ask yourself the following questions:

- **Why is the information familiar?** Just because information comes to mind easily, that doesn't always mean it is accurate. You now know you're more likely to trust information that you've heard multiple times, that you can be susceptible to the influences of misinformation, and that you can generate erroneous information when it's consistent with the *gist* of an event. So, before you act on the information coming to mind, take a moment to evaluate why that content is springing to your consciousness. You may realize it's likely a false memory.
- **Could it have happened that way?** Take a moment to think about the details you recall about the memory. Are they consistent with one another? Or is one detail mutually exclusive of another (such as cousin Suzy and your daughter both being at the same Thanksgiving dinner). This is a strategy called *recall-to-reject*;[15] as the wording implies, the recall of one piece of information from your memory can help you to reject some other information as being a false memory.
- **How well should you remember this content?** If someone tells you you've eaten at a neighborhood restaurant before, you might accept their claim as true if you eat out a lot and, after a while, the meals all blur together. But if you would have dined at the restaurant in question only on a special occasion, then you probably should suggest to the person that they may have you confused for someone else. In other words, if an event would have been *distinctive*, then you should be more likely to take the *lack* of a strong memory as evidence that it didn't occur.

Part 3

WHEN THERE IS TOO LITTLE MEMORY—OR TOO MUCH

13

Just normal aging— or is it Alzheimer's disease?

"I'm so worried about my memory," says the 82-year-old accountant and mother of three. "All of my friends are having memory
problems. Many of them have dementia, and some even have
Alzheimer's disease. I think I'm getting it too—I know I am. This
morning I walked into my bedroom and could not remember what
I was looking for—not until I walked back down to the chilly base-
ment and remembered the sweater I had gone to get. And coming
up with people's names, forget it! If I don't see someone regularly,
I have a terrible time recalling their name. That's not all. Last week,
I was driving to the bank while my son was telling me about the
grandchildren—they're all doing so well—and the next thing I know
I'm in the parking lot of the grocery store. I had no recollection of
the driving for the last 10 minutes nor how I ended up at the grocery store instead of the bank."

Is this 82-year-old accountant developing Alzheimer's disease
or aging normally? In this chapter we will review the changes
in memory that occur with normal aging as well as brain disorders of aging such as Alzheimer's disease so that you will be
able to tell them apart. We'll also discuss how you can use the

other memory systems that are relatively intact to compensate for some of the memory problems that occur in normal aging and various brain disorders.

NORMAL AGING

Individuals who are aging normally in their 60s, 70s, and 80s experience some difficulty keeping information in mind in their working memory (see Chapter 3). They also need to use more effort to learn new information and to retrieve information when they need it from their episodic memory (see Chapter 4), and they have trouble recalling people's names from their semantic memory (see Chapter 5). Experiencing these memory challenges with increased frequency as you age does not need to be cause for alarm. We'll examine these difficulties, and then turn to procedural memory (see Chapter 2), which is relatively preserved in aging.

Older Frontal Lobes

Memory difficulties in normal aging often are related to changes that occur to the frontal lobes and their connections to the rest of the brain. Older frontal lobes just don't function as well as they did when they were younger. Some researchers and clinicians believe this is due to a small amount of age-related damage to this part of the brain and its connections from tiny strokes or other pathology (we'll review strokes later on in this chapter). Other researchers believe these changes to the frontal lobes are due to normal, physiologic changes not related to a disorder, such as an alteration in the prevalence of brain cell receptors that facilitates the stabilization of memories at the cost of diminishing the ability to form new memories.

Working Memory in Normal Aging

Recall that the prefrontal cortex is the *central executive* of the working memory system. Since frontal lobe function decreases with aging, it should not surprise you that older adults show diminished working memory abilities relative to younger adults. Compared to those in their 20s and 30s, older adults generally cannot keep as much information in mind or manipulate it as easily. This means that, compared to when they were younger, older adults are usually slower to add up a column of numbers in their head and less able to keep in mind a map of a city they are visiting for the first time.

Episodic Memory in Normal Aging

There are three major changes that occur in episodic memory as people age, all related to their diminished frontal lobe function. We'll consider them each in turn, along with some simple measures you can take to compensate for these changes.

First, it takes more effort to pay attention and thus to get the desired information into episodic memory. Simply repeating information, however, can help you overcome this difficulty. So, try repeating your shopping list, an address you are driving to, or the day's agenda a couple of times in order to remember them.

Second, it takes more time, effort—and often some strategies—to get the desired information out of episodic memory. With diminished frontal lobe function, your ability to search through your episodic memory to find and rebuild the memory you're looking for is diminished. Sometimes just concentrating hard and giving yourself a bit of time is enough for the desired memory to come to mind. At other times you will need to use strategies to bring the desired memory to mind. Try to recall the location in which the memory was formed— that cue might trigger recall of the memory. See Chapter 9 and Part 5 for many more suggestions on how to improve your memory retrieval.

Third, older adults are more likely to experience a mixed-up, distorted, or outright false memory. Although these types of memory mix-ups can happen to anyone, because frontal lobe function declines as we age, false memories are more likely to occur to older adults. As we discussed in Chapter 12, you can reduce false memories by paying close attention to the details of information when you are learning them and trying again to picture as many specific details as you can when you are retrieving the information.

Semantic Memory in Normal Aging

Most healthy older adults experience some difficulty retrieving people's names or the titles of books or movies. There are two reasons for this difficulty. The first is their frontal lobe dysfunction. It is your frontal lobes that help you search through your stores of semantic knowledge to retrieve the specific information you're looking for. So, because of frontal lobe dysfunction, it may be more difficult for older adults to retrieve any type of knowledge. But why are people's names specifically difficult for older adults? We believe it is likely related to the shrinkage that so often occurs in aging to the tip of the temporal lobe—the very place where the names of people are usually stored. One way to improve your retrieval of people's names is to think about other things you know about the individual: their occupation, hobbies, family, appearance, and so forth. See Chapter 24 for additional suggestions on how to improve your retrieval of names.

Procedural Memory in Normal Aging

One aspect of memory that is generally preserved in individuals who are aging normally is procedural memory, the ability to learn and use skills and habits. This means that if you always wanted to take up golf (or baseball or snowshoeing) but never had the time while you were working, and you are now retired and in your 60s, 70s, or 80s, there is no reason that you cannot take lessons and begin to learn the new sport. Just remember that, like any activity at any age, it may take a number of years of practice before you are proficient (hopefully a little sooner for snowshoeing).

Equally if not more importantly, you can also use your procedural memory to compensate for difficulties in your episodic memory. For example, perhaps when you were younger you could leave your keys anywhere and always be able to find them. Now that you're older, you notice that you're hunting around the house for your keys daily. If you use your procedural memory to train yourself to get into the habit of always leaving your keys in the same place, you'll always be able to find them when you need them.

UPSIDES TO AN AGING MEMORY SYSTEM

Although older adults often notice their increased memory difficulties, there are also benefits to the way that older adults' brains record information. While younger adults' brains may be drafting memory structures with lots of details—some of them unimportant—older adults' memory structures are more likely to include just the essential elements. Remembering just the critical information can make it easier for older adults to avoid the common pitfall of "missing the forest for the trees," allowing them to grasp the overall importance of a situation. The way older adults' brains build memory structures can also make it easier for them to see commonalities between different situations and to understand how knowledge acquired in one context can be applied to the situation at hand. In fact, some of the wisdom that comes with aging may be attributable to changes in the way the aging brain builds its memory structures.

WHEN IT'S NOT NORMAL AGING

Now that you have a better understanding of the changes in memory that occur with normal aging, we're going to turn to understanding memory loss. Keep in mind that when older individuals develop a brain disease affecting thinking and memory, they will typically experience all the changes that occur in normal aging *plus* the changes that come with the brain disease.

MEMORY LOSS TERMINOLOGY

The terminology used by clinicians and researchers to describe memory loss and the individuals who have it can be quite confusing. In this section we will describe the general syndromes that can apply to many underlying brain problems (such as dementia, mild cognitive impairment, and subjective cognitive decline, progressing from most to least severe), and then we'll dive into the specific brain disorders (such as Alzheimer's disease, vascular dementia, and frontotemporal dementia) in the next section.

Dementia

Dementia is not a diagnosis in and of itself. Dementia is a term that means an individual has experienced progressive decline in their thinking and memory severe enough to interfere with day-to-day function. Dementia is considered to be mild if the individual has difficulty only with somewhat complicated daily activities, such as paying bills, shopping, preparing meals, or taking medicines. If the individual has difficulties with more basic activities of daily living, such as dressing, bathing, eating, or using the toilet, the dementia is considered to be in the moderate or severe stage. Most people with dementia become more impaired over time, depending on the cause. Different causes of dementia affect different brain regions, producing different symptoms (see Figure 13.1).

Mild Cognitive Impairment

We use the term *mild cognitive impairment* when (1) a decline in thinking and/or memory has been noticed by the individual,

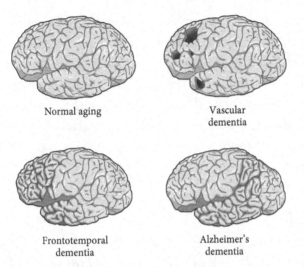

Normal aging

Vascular
dementia

Frontotemporal
dementia

Alzheimer's
dementia

Figure 13.1. A small amount of brain shrinkage occurs in normal aging. Parietal and temporal regions shrink in Alzheimer's dementia. Frontal and temporal regions shrink in frontotemporal dementia. Strokes damage the brain in vascular dementia.

their family, or their doctor, (2) impairment—typically mild— is present on tests of thinking and/or memory, and (3) their daily function is essentially normal, although activities may require a bit more effort. Note that because their daily function is essentially normal, by definition individuals with mild cognitive impairment do not have dementia. Research suggests that approximately half of people with mild cognitive impairment end up declining over time and developing dementia at a rate of about 5% to 15% per year, whereas the other half remain stable—or actually improve.

Subjective Cognitive Decline

Some individuals are concerned enough about their memory function to see their doctor, but their performance on tests of thinking and memory is normal, as is their daily function. These individuals have *subjective cognitive decline*. Most people with subjective cognitive decline are simply worried about their memories and there is actually nothing wrong with them. There are some people, however, who have noticed a slight but real decline in their thinking or memory despite their performance being normal on standard cognitive tests. For this reason, when compared to individuals without concerns about their memory, a few people with subjective cognitive decline are somewhat more likely to end up with a diagnosable memory disorder over the next 5 to 10 years.

ALZHEIMER'S DISEASE

In 1907, Alois Alzheimer described the case of a 51-year-old woman he observed in the insane asylum of Frankfurt am Main. "Her memory is seriously impaired," he wrote. "If objects are shown to her, she names them correctly, but almost immediately afterwards she has forgotten everything."[1] He goes on to describe what he saw in her brain under the microscope after her death, including the neurofibrillary tangles, "only a tangle of fibrils indicates the place where a neuron was previously located," and amyloid plaques, "minute miliary foci which are caused by deposition of a special substance in the cortex." Although this brief description in Alzheimer's own words (translated from German) concisely summarizes this disease of memory caused by tangles and plaques, we'll expand a bit regarding the common memory deficits observed.

Memory Loss Progresses but Awareness Diminishes

Because Alzheimer's disease progresses slowly over about 4 to 12 years, most individuals with Alzheimer's will go through the mild cognitive impairment stage before they develop dementia, as do individuals with other causes of dementia. Some individuals will experience subjective cognitive decline prior to mild cognitive impairment. Once function is impaired and

Alzheimer's disease dementia is diagnosed, the disease progresses from the mild to the moderate and then to the severe
stage. In the mild cognitive impairment and mild dementia
stages, individuals with Alzheimer's are often very aware of their
disease and distressed by their memory problems. However, as
the disease progresses, individuals with Alzheimer's generally
forget that they cannot remember and so become unaware that
anything is wrong with them.

Alzheimer's Plus Aging

Because most people with Alzheimer's are in their 60s, 70s,
or 80s, the cognitive deficits observed in most individuals
with this disease are really caused by Alzheimer's tangles and
plaques *plus* normal aging. This means that most individuals with Alzheimer's disease have all of the memory problems
described earlier in the section on normal aging, *plus* the additional problems that we will now describe.

Rapid Forgetting

The episodic memory deficit that is most characteristic of
Alzheimer's is *rapid forgetting*. That is, even when information is repeated while it is being learned, and even when
hints and cues are given when it is trying to be retrieved, the
memory cannot be reassembled—because the information
is rapidly forgotten. This rapid forgetting is directly related
to where Alzheimer's disease strikes first and foremost—the
inner part of the temporal lobe, including the hippocampus. Because the hippocampus and related structures are
damaged, new memories for events will be impaired, new
information will be learned with difficulty or not at all, and
retrieval of memory for recent events and recently learned
information will be impaired. Older, consolidated memories
for events, however, can often be retrieved—although they
will lack the vividness and subjective experience of a true

episodic memory. See Chapter 4 and Part 2 for more information on these topics.

Rapid forgetting leads to several characteristic problems in daily life. Because they have difficulty remembering where they put things, individuals with Alzheimer's often lose items such as their keys, glasses, wallet, purse, and mobile phone. Because they don't recall conversations, individuals with Alzheimer's frequently tell the same stories to the same people repeatedly, and they ask the same questions again and again and again—sometimes many times in an hour. Because they have difficulty recalling the route they have traveled and remembering landmarks while walking or driving, individuals with Alzheimer's often get lost, even on familiar routes. As the disease progresses, they begin to lose track of the day, date, month, season, and year, because they cannot retain this information.

False Memories

False memories are common in individuals with Alzheimer's disease. Sometimes it is simply a matter of believing a memory that occurred 30 years ago happened today—such as a conversation with a long-deceased parent. Or perhaps misremembering that they took their medications today when they took it yesterday. Sometimes the false memory may be more outlandish, such as combining events they heard on television with aspects of their own life. We have had patients tell us about a trip they took to an exotic country—only to later find out that they mixed their memory for a television program with that of a local day trip they took.

Word-Finding Difficulties

The semantic memory deficit that is most characteristic of Alzheimer's disease is difficulty retrieving not only people's names, but common, ordinary words used in everyday life, such as umbrella, closet, bookcase, and photograph. This impairment is so common and pervasive that family members typically get into the habit of jumping in to provide the missing word when their loved ones with the disease pause, searching for words. The semantic deficit in Alzheimer's is more extensive than in normal aging because the damage from Alzheimer's involves large portions of the outer part of the temporal lobe.

Habits and Routines Are Relatively Preserved

Procedural memory is fairly intact in mild Alzheimer's disease. Habits and routines are therefore relatively preserved and can be used, to some extent, to compensate for episodic memory impairments. For example, if an individual with Alzheimer's has difficulty remembering what is on the agenda for the day, rather than asking five times an hour they may be able to get into the habit of looking at a daily planner on the refrigerator, which they can do as often as they wish. Individuals with mild Alzheimer's can also learn to routinely use memory aids, such as taking medications from a pillbox and writing things down in a notebook as soon as someone tells them something they need to remember, such as an appointment. Medications that increase the chemical acetylcholine in the brain can also help improve memory (for example, donepezil [Aricept]).

VASCULAR COGNITIVE IMPAIRMENT AND VASCULAR DEMENTIA

A type of memory impairment with a different root cause is *vascular cognitive impairment*, the term used when memory and thinking are impaired due to strokes. If the impairment is severe enough to interfere with daily function, we use the term *vascular dementia*.

Most strokes occur when an artery sending blood from the heart to the brain becomes blocked off; that part of the brain doesn't receive enough blood and dies. We used the word "vascular" to emphasize that the problem is with the blood vessels. Individuals are at risk for strokes if they are over age 55, have had prior strokes or stroke warning signs (called *transient ischemic attacks* or *TIAs*), were or are smokers, drink more than one alcoholic beverage per day, lead a sedentary lifestyle, eat an unhealthy diet, or have heart disease, diabetes, high cholesterol, high blood pressure, obesity, or disease in other blood vessels of the body.

Large strokes are generally noticeable to individuals and their family, as they may cause sudden loss of vision or speech, sudden weakness or numbness of an arm or a leg, or sudden impairment in coordination or walking. Small strokes, however, typically show no outward signs and are only noticeable over years as first dozens and then hundreds of them accumulate in the brain. Luckily, most strokes are small.

Damage to the Brain's Wiring

Although strokes can literally affect any area of the brain, most affect the "white matter" that makes up the brain's wiring—the connections between the brain cells—rather than the information-processing part of the brain cells. Because most of the wiring in the brain goes to and from the frontal lobes, vascular cognitive impairment causes frontal lobe dysfunction. Thinking is also generally slower, as brain processes have to work around roadblocks due to strokes.

Like Normal Aging—Only More So

Because vascular cognitive impairment tends to cause frontal lobe dysfunction, it leads to many of the same problems observed in normal aging, but to a greater extent. Working memory is diminished and it will be difficult for these individuals to keep information in their mind and manipulate it. Episodic memory problems include difficulty getting the desired information into memory, needing more effort to get the information out of memory, and frequently experiencing false and distorted memories.

Different Than Alzheimer's Disease

Because the memory problems in vascular cognitive impairment are due to frontal lobe dysfunction, the memory loss manifests somewhat differently compared to that of Alzheimer's disease. In general, there is no rapid forgetting. This means that in vascular cognitive impairment repetition will enable information to be learned. As orienting information, such as the date, is generally observed repeatedly during the day through newspapers, radio, television, and conversations, these individuals are usually oriented to the day, date, month, season, and year. They generally don't repeat questions and stories. It is difficult for them to retrieve previously learned information spontaneously but—in contrast to Alzheimer's—hints and cues help tremendously such that most information can be retrieved with the right cue. Although there are some difficulties retrieving semantic information, word-finding difficulties are less prominent compared to Alzheimer's.

Procedural memory governing habits and routines may or may not be intact in vascular cognitive impairment depending on where the strokes are in the brain. Strokes often affect the basal ganglia and cerebellum, two of the key brain structures needed for procedural memory.

FRONTOTEMPORAL DEMENTIA

In behavioral variant frontotemporal dementia, the frontal lobes are directly damaged by pathology (of which there are many types). Marked changes in behavior and personality are the most prominent features, often including socially inappropriate behavior, loss of sympathy or empathy, compulsive or ritualistic behavior, and binge eating (particularly of sweets).

Depending upon where in the frontal lobes the damage occurs, individuals with this disorder may show relatively normal memory or they may manifest all the problems described in patients with vascular cognitive impairment. When they have memory problems it tends to be difficult to improve them because individuals with this disorder generally refuse to believe that there is anything wrong with them. Instead, the family needs to adapt to them.

NORMAL PRESSURE HYDROCEPHALUS

In normal pressure hydrocephalus (despite the name) there is a problem with the movement of spinal fluid in and around the brain such that the ventricular system inside the brain enlarges and pushes on the brain's wiring that runs beside these expanding ventricles. This pressure can damage the wiring and produce memory problems similar to individuals with vascular cognitive impairment, in addition to incontinence and difficulty walking. The definitive treatment is with a tube to drain off some of the fluid.

PARKINSON'S DISEASE, PARKINSON'S DISEASE DEMENTIA, AND DEMENTIA WITH LEWY BODIES

Individuals with Parkinson's disease, Parkinson's disease dementia, and dementia with Lewy bodies have a reduction of the chemical dopamine in the basal ganglia of the brain, which generally produces stiff and slow movements, tremor, and impairment in procedural memory. These individuals therefore experience difficulty in learning new skills, habits, and routines.

Frontal lobe function is also impaired when there is a loss of dopamine in the basal ganglia, and thus individuals with these disorders can manifest memory problems similar to those with vascular cognitive impairment.

PRIMARY PROGRESSIVE APHASIA AND SEMANTIC DEMENTIA

Individuals with primary progressive aphasia have problems with language that interfere with their daily function. This disorder has several different variants, and difficulty accessing words from semantic memory is prominent in all of them. Individuals with the *logopenic* variant experience difficulty in retrieving common, ordinary words like hammock, vase, or blanket. Individuals with the *non-fluent/agrammatic* variant experience those word-finding difficulties plus halting, effortful speech that is missing other words as well. As discussed in Chapter 5, those with the *semantic* variant not only experience word-finding problems but may also lose what some words mean, such that given a specific word (such as "vase") they may or may not be able to describe what its meaning is. Lastly, individuals with the related disorder of *semantic dementia* not only lose the meaning of some specific words but also lose the meaning of the items themselves such that they can no longer use them—as if they grew up in a culture that simply didn't have hammocks or vases.

LOOKING FOR MORE INFORMATION?

Want to know more about these topics? Andrew and his colleague Maureen K. O'Connor have written two entire books on memory loss in normal aging, Alzheimer's disease, and dementia. For individuals with mild memory problems, we recommend *Seven Steps to Managing Your Aging Memory: What's Normal, What's Not, and What to Do About It*.[2] For individuals caring for their loved ones with dementia in the moderate or severe stages, we recommend *Six Steps to Managing Alzheimer's Disease and Dementia: A Guide for Families.*[3]

Lastly, what about our 82-year-old accountant introduced at the beginning of the chapter? Although we cannot say she is aging normally without a proper evaluation, the problems she shared with us are not concerning. It is normal to walk into a room, become distracted by something else, and forget the reason why you are there. As mentioned earlier in this chapter, it is common for healthy older adults to have difficulty recalling people's names. And if you multitask while driving you might very well end up in the wrong place and have no recollection of how you got there, because you are not paying enough attention to where you are going.

CHANGES IN MEMORY FROM AGING AND COMMON BRAIN DISORDERS IN LATE LIFE

Let's review the common ways that one's memory changes with age in health and disease:

- Normal aging
  - More effort is needed to get information into memory.
  - More time and effort are needed to retrieve memories.
  - False memories are more common.
  - Trouble retrieving names of people, places, books, and movies is common.
  - Remembering just the essential elements may lead to wisdom.
- Terminology for memory disorders
  - *Dementia* means there is cognitive impairment severe enough to interfere with day-to-day function.
  - *Mild cognitive impairment* is when cognitive problems are noticeable, present on tests, but mild enough so that day-to-day function is preserved.

  ○ *Subjective cognitive decline* is used when individuals are concerned about their cognition but they score normally on tests of thinking and memory and function normally as well.
- Alzheimer's disease
  ○ *Rapid forgetting* of information is common.
  ○ *False memories* are common.
  ○ *Word-finding difficulties* are often present even for ordinary nouns.
- Vascular cognitive impairment and vascular dementia
  ○ Thinking and memory processes are slowed.
  ○ More effort is needed to get information into memory.
  ○ More effort is needed to retrieve memories.

14

What else can go wrong with your memory?

A 32-year-old man was brought to the hospital by his girlfriend for confusion. Previously healthy other than occasional migraine head-aches, she reported that he keeps asking her, "What's going on?" and "What are we doing?" every 5 minutes, despite her repeat-edly explaining everything to him. When asked what he was doing before the spell came on, she looked at the floor and then, some-what embarrassed, explained that they had engaged in a lengthy lovemaking session right before the spell started. Upon examina-tion, although the man's working memory was normal and so he could keep information in mind, if he was distracted for a few sec-onds he would forget everything related to his visit to the hospital, such as not remembering meeting the doctor minutes before. He also did not recall his lovemaking session with his girlfriend—or, indeed, anything else that happened that day.

What is going on with this 32-year-old man? Is he having a seizure? Did he have a stroke? Is he having a psychological reac-tion related to his sexual activity? Or perhaps he is having a side effect from a pleasure-enhancing medication that he took?

To determine what happened with this young man, we will now turn to some of the common medical, neurologic, and psychiatric disorders that can cause memory difficulties in individuals of any age. We will begin with one of the most common reversible causes of memory problems: medication side effects. (Note that, unless otherwise specified, in this chapter the term "memory" refers to episodic memory.)

MEDICATION SIDE EFFECTS

The development of modern medications has dramatically changed our ability to treat many disorders. Unfortunately, most medications have side effects, sometimes including effects on memory. In this section we will review those classes of medications that may impair memory, and briefly explain why the medications have those side effects. The Appendix has many more medications by name; skim it to see if any of your medications could be impairing your memory.

Note that it is important to consult your doctor prior to stopping or changing the dose of any of your medications. Often the benefits of the primary, intended use of the medication outweigh the side effects. Although the side effects of many medications can be dramatically reduced by lowering the dose, some medications must be lowered slowly or serious complications—such as seizures—may occur.

WHY DO MEDICATIONS AFFECT MEMORY?

Medications that affect memory do so by altering the chemical messengering systems in the brain. You can imagine these messengering systems as sets of locks and keys: A particular chemical serves as a key that can unlock the function of a neighboring brain cell, so long as that cell has a type of lock that the key can open. In these cases, the chemical key is referred to as a *neurotransmitter* and the lock is referred to as a *receptor*. Typically, for each neurotransmitter there are a few different types (and subtypes) of receptors, sometimes needing different amounts of the neurotransmitter in order for them to unlock. These receptors are often distributed across many parts of the brain, and sometimes they exist in other parts of the body as well. Usually, a medication is being prescribed because of its effects in a specific part of the brain or body, or because of its effects on one particular type of receptor. But sometimes, the medication affects not only the desired parts of the brain or body or the desired receptor types, but also other brain regions and receptor types. In some of these latter instances, this "off-target action" can lead the medications to impair memory. Here, we briefly describe the neurotransmitter systems that are most likely to be implicated when medications cause memory disruptions, and outline some of the common reasons why medications affecting those systems are prescribed.

THE CHOLINERGIC SYSTEM

Acetylcholine is a molecule that acts as a neurotransmitter; neurons that produce acetylcholine are found throughout the brain, and there are two primary types of locks (receptors) to which it can bind. One of these types of receptors is found in large numbers in the cells within the hippocampus and in cells that communicate with the hippocampus. Given the critical role that the hippocampus plays in memory, it is therefore not surprising that medications that disrupt these cholinergic locks-and-keys tend to impair memory. The two most common types of medications that affect memory via actions on the cholinergic system are anticholinergic antidepressants and medications for dizziness and incontinence.

Anticholinergic Medications: Older Antidepressants and Treatments for Dizziness and Incontinence

Most currently prescribed antidepressants are safe, with few side effects. The ones that do cause memory problems are those that are anticholinergic. As the prefix *anti-* indicates, this category of antidepressant works by disrupting the cholinergic system. This disruption can be helpful for treating symptoms of depression, but it can also cause memory impairments; these medications can sometimes cause drowsiness and confusion as well.

Anticholinergic medications also are often prescribed for treatment of dizziness and vertigo. Short-term use of these medications to relieve symptoms, such as those caused by an inner ear infection or from being on a boat, is typically fine. But taking these medications for more than a day or two can lead to memory impairments.

Because acetylcholine also works to activate muscles, many of the medications that treat bladder incontinence or muscle spasms are anticholinergic and can have memory side effects. Bladder incontinence leading to urinary accidents is a serious problem that may make it difficult for people to go out in public, and if you or a loved one has incontinence and are taking a medication that works to stop or greatly diminish accidents, we recommend continuing it. However, many people take incontinence medications without a noticeable reduction in accidents. If this is the case, we recommend speaking with the doctor to see if it can be reduced, eliminated, or replaced with one that works as well or better with fewer side effects.

THE HISTAMINE SYSTEM

Histamine, like other neurotransmitters, acts as a key in our lock-and-key analogy, but the locks it opens often serve to modulate other neurotransmitter systems. You might imagine histamine as not only opening some of its own locks but also partly opening other locks, so that they are easier for the other neurotransmitter keys to open. This can lead histamine to have widespread effects throughout the brain, with some research framing the role of histamine as being a regulator of overall brain activity levels.[1] Histamine also has a specific role in memory, with a high density of its receptors in the hippocampus and amygdala.[2]

Antihistamines for Allergies, Cold and Flu Symptoms, Sleep Aids, and Vertigo

Given the role of histamine in regulating overall levels of brain activity, it is perhaps not surprising that *antihistamine* medications, which work by blocking histamine's actions, often cause drowsiness and confusion. The drowsiness can in itself be disruptive to memory by reducing attentional focus. Antihistamines can also affect memory more directly, likely via their effects within the hippocampus and neighboring structures in the medial temporal lobe. Many older allergy medications as well as common cold and flu remedies, nighttime pain relievers, and over-the-counter sleeping pills are antihistamines. Antihistamines are also often prescribed for motion sickness and to reduce dizziness and vertigo.

THE DOPAMINE SYSTEM AND ANTIPSYCHOTICS

Dopamine is another neurotransmitter that is essential for the function of neural pathways important for motor behavior as well as for reward processing and decision-making. In fact, dopamine is critical to the proper functioning of both the prefrontal cortex and the hippocampus.

Problems arise when there is too little dopamine in the brain, leading to diseases such as Parkinson's, and also when there is too much—an overactive dopamine system is thought to underlie the hallucinations and delusions experienced during psychosis. Thus, to treat the latter types of symptoms, many antipsychotics—especially the older, so-called typical antipsychotics—work to reduce dopamine transmission. Although these antipsychotics were developed to treat adults with schizophrenia or mania, they are often prescribed for individuals with dementia with difficult behaviors. Because these medications disrupt the dopamine system, memory impairment in individuals of any age is common with these medications. Note that the newer, "atypical" antipsychotics often work via other neurotransmitter systems and are less likely to affect memory.

GAMMA-AMINOBUTYRIC ACID (GABA) AND THE BENZODIAZEPINES

GABA is an amino acid, one of the building blocks of proteins. It is also one of the most widely distributed neurotransmitters in the brain. In the nervous system, it serves as an inhibitory neurotransmitter, so rather than increasing the activity of the cells with which it communicates, it decreases their activity.

Decreased action of GABA has been associated with anxiety and other psychiatric disorders. Therefore, unlike the medications we have discussed previously that work by reducing the actions of neurotransmitter systems, the goal of GABA medications is to *increase* the action of GABA in the brain. Unfortunately, when GABA is raised to the levels needed to be beneficial for anxiety and related conditions, it is typically disruptive to memory. Thus, benzodiazepines—one class of medications that increase the action of GABA and are often used to treat anxiety—almost always cause memory impairment, drowsiness, and confusion. In fact, when doctors perform a medical procedure but don't want you to remember it (such as a colonoscopy), this is the class of medication they give you. Note that any reduction or stopping of these medications should always be done under the supervision of your doctor; seizures may occur if they are stopped abruptly.

OTHER MEDICATIONS WITH MEMORY SIDE EFFECTS

The Appendix lists many more medications that can affect memory. These include seizure medications, tremor medications, sleeping medications, narcotic medications used to relieve pain, and some of the medications to treat migraines.

Keep in mind that herbal remedies are just another type of medication with their own side effects; they are not intrinsically safer just because they are herbal. Herbal medications can influence multiple neurotransmitter systems. Many cause memory impairment and some also cause nervousness, fatigue, dizziness, or confusion.

A note on sleeping medications: Sleep is critically important for memory for a number of reasons (which we review in Chapter 20), and it might therefore seem wise to take medication to help you sleep. The problem, however, is that the vast majority of sleeping medications do not help you to get a restorative night of sleep; they act more like sedatives, depriving you of many of the benefits of healthy sleep. They are generally antihistamines, benzodiazepines, or benzodiazepine-like substances, all of which may impair your memory. If you must intervene pharmacologically, melatonin and acetaminophen are the two best options; otherwise, as discussed in Chapter 20, we recommend nonpharmacological treatments for sleep problems.

REGULATION OF MEMORY BY VITAMINS AND HORMONES

There are a variety of medical disorders that can affect memory. Two of the most common are vitamin deficiencies and thyroid disorders, so everyone with memory concerns should ensure they do not have a vitamin- or thyroid-related disorder.

Vitamin Deficiencies Can Impair Memory

Low levels of vitamin B_{12} (cyanocobalamin) can cause a number of medical problems, including impairment of memory and thinking. If you have noticed memory or thinking problems, we recommend that you get your B_{12} level checked. Note that although sometimes the B_{12} deficiency is due to not getting enough of the vitamin from your diet, more often it is due to problems absorbing the vitamin. That's why even if you are taking vitamin B_{12} supplements, it's important to check your levels.

Although your body can make vitamin D when your skin is exposed to sunlight, many people have vitamin D deficiency. Such a deficiency has not been proven to cause memory loss, but a strong correlation has been found between low vitamin D levels and dementia. We therefore recommend either having your vitamin D levels checked or asking your doctor if taking the standard dose of 2,000 IU of vitamin D_3 (cholecalciferol) daily would be right for you.

Thiamine (vitamin B_1) deficiency can cause a form of potentially reversible memory loss and confusion called Wernicke's encephalopathy, as well as a devastating, permanent loss of memory called Korsakoff syndrome (or Korsakoff amnesia). In developed countries thiamine deficiency and these disorders are typically associated with alcoholism. However, in other parts of the world it may be associated with poor nutrition. Thiamine pills are available over the counter, and thiamine-rich foods include whole grains, legumes, pork, fruit, and yeast.

Thyroid Disorders Can Impair Memory

Abnormal thyroid hormone levels in your body can cause impaired memory as well as difficulty concentrating, irritability, mood instability, restlessness, and confusion. A simple blood test can screen for it, so you should ask your doctor about it if you are experiencing memory problems.

Hormonal Changes During Menopause

Many middle-aged women notice a change in their memory at about the time they are beginning to go through menopause. The scientific literature is unclear, however, whether the menopausal changes in estrogen and progesterone are causing the changes in memory, or whether it is an aging-related effect that is not specifically tied to those hormonal changes; many individuals (including men) experience memory changes in middle age. What is clear is that hormone replacement therapy in postmenopausal women does not help memory nor does it reduce the risk of memory problems in the future.

BODILY STRESS, INFECTIONS, AND DISEASES AFFECT MEMORY

There are many reasons why, when something is wrong in the body, there can be consequences for memory. Sometimes, the effects are indirect: For instance, the body may release stress hormones when injured or fighting an infection, and those hormones may trigger a cascade of processes that have consequences for memory function. Other times, the problems in the body can have more direct effects on the brain. Although there is a protective blood–brain barrier—acting like a wall of defense to keep pathogens (such as viruses and bacteria) that may infect the rest of the body from entering the brain—the barrier is imperfect, and sometimes pathogens cross into the brain, leading to inflammation that can impact thinking and memory. The bottom line is that the function of the brain will be influenced by what is happening in the rest of the body.

Lyme Disease and Other Chronic Infections

There are many chronic infections that can cause trouble with memory and thinking, including diseases spread by ticks such as Lyme disease and Rocky Mountain spotted fever. If you live in an area where these or other such diseases are common and you spend time outdoors in the woods or you have found a tick on you, you should speak with your doctor about getting tested for one of these treatable diseases.

These tickborne diseases are just two of the many other treatable infectious diseases that can interfere with memory. If you are having any symptoms of infection such as fever, cough, night sweats, chills, or muscle aches, you should see your doctor right away to find out if you have a treatable infection (not just because of its effects on your memory!).

Finally, if you think it is possible that you have contracted a sexually transmitted disease, make sure you mention it to your doctor as soon as possible. Two sexually transmitted diseases, syphilis and HIV/AIDS, may first become noticeable because of thinking and memory difficulties. Both of these disorders may damage the brain directly or, in the case of HIV, lead to other so-called opportunistic infections in the brain.

Encephalitis

Encephalitis involves an inflammation of the brain, usually caused by an infection of brain tissue itself. The most common cause of encephalitis is the herpes simplex virus, the same virus that causes cold sores in the mouth. For reasons that we don't fully understand, in rare cases the virus travels through the nerves in the mouth or the nose to their origins in the temporal lobes and begins to attack the brain. Because the inside of the temporal lobe is home to the hippocampus and the lower, outside aspect of temporal lobe is home to semantic memory, this type of encephalitis may produce a devastating impairment of both episodic and semantic memory.

Coronavirus Disease 2019 (COVID-19)

Have you heard the term "brain fog" being used in relation to COVID-19 infection? Brain fog is not a medical or scientific term; it is a term used by individuals to describe how they feel when their thinking is sluggish, fuzzy, and not sharp. COVID-19 infections may cause brain fog by damaging the brain in several ways—each of which can lead to memory and thinking impairments. First, it can infect the brain directly, causing encephalitis (inflammation of the brain). Second, it is a risk factor for strokes. Third, because it frequently infects the lungs, COVID-19 can deprive the brain of oxygen. In addition to these very serious problems, many individuals who were thought to have fully recovered from COVID-19 infection have persistent impairment in working memory,[3] which leads to difficulties remembering new episodic and semantic information as well. Lastly, a group of German and American doctors have speculated that the combination of the direct infection with the virus, systemic inflammation, increased risk of strokes, and damage to lungs and other bodily organs might place survivors of COVID-19 at increased risk for Alzheimer's disease in the future.[4] It is too early to tell if this speculation is correct, but we hope not.

Diabetes

Diabetes can cause memory impairment in several different ways. First, diabetes is a risk factor for strokes, and strokes can cause memory problems, as described later in this chapter. Second, when the levels of blood sugar rise too high or fall too low, there can be periods of memory loss and confusion. Lastly, the hippocampus and other parts of the brain can be permanently damaged if the control of diabetes is too strict and blood sugar concentrations repeatedly drop to dangerously low levels.

Hospitalizations, Major Surgeries, and Anesthesia

Many people can become confused and delirious and experience memory problems when they are hospitalized for any serious medical problem or a major surgery, such as a life-threatening infection or a hip surgery. Sometimes the memory problems are related to the powerful medications that are given at the time, as described earlier in this chapter and in the Appendix. Other times, they are related to the effects of the stress that the body is under and the hormonal cascades triggered by those stress responses. As the individual recovers and the effects of the medications wear off, the memory should return to normal.

Sometimes the confusion and memory problems are related to anesthesia, which brings up a question we are frequently asked: Does general anesthesia cause long-lasting memory impairment or dementia? Our review of the available medical literature suggests that general anesthesia, properly administered, does not cause permanent memory impairment or dementia. It may, however, cause delirium (confusion), making a hospitalization prolonged and unpleasant. It may also bring out symptoms of memory loss in an individual when these symptoms were not yet apparent in daily life. For these last two reasons, we generally recommend that local or spinal anesthesia be used whenever the surgeon and anesthesiologist feel it is safe to do so. If, however, there is any question about the individual moving around during a delicate surgical procedure, then general anesthesia will be the safest method.

Organ Failure

It shouldn't be surprising to hear that, in order for your brain to function properly, all of your other organs need to function properly as well. So, if you or a loved one are experiencing serious problems with the liver, kidney, heart, or lungs, the brain won't be able to function properly, and memory impairment will likely be present. If the bodily organs recover, brain and memory function will return to normal in most cases.

NEUROLOGIC DISORDERS

Here we will describe some of the common brain disorders that cause memory problems. Chapter 13 has already presented dementia, mild cognitive impairment, subjective cognitive decline, Alzheimer's disease, vascular cognitive impairment, vascular dementia, frontotemporal dementia, normal pressure hydrocephalus, Parkinson's disease, Parkinson's disease dementia, dementia with Lewy bodies, primary progressive aphasia, and semantic dementia and the memory problems associated with each.

Brain Tumors

Brain tumors generally cause memory problems in one of three ways. First, some tumors will directly invade and destroy one of the brain's memory centers such as the hippocampus (for episodic memory), the cerebellum (for procedural memory), or their connections. Second, some tumors, such as those found in a brain structure above the nose called the *pituitary gland*, may disrupt thyroid hormone or other brain chemicals important for memory. Third, because they are growing inside the confined space of the skull, many tumors—even benign ones that are not cancerous—will compress one of the brain's memory centers or their connections. Because tumors can cause memory loss, a brain scan looking for them is part of the standard evaluation of memory impairment.

Epilepsy and Seizures

Epilepsy and seizures can impair memory in two different ways. First, although most seizures involve complete loss of consciousness, rhythmic jerking of arms and legs, and bladder incontinence, some seizures are subtle and only manifest with a slight alteration of consciousness. These *focal impaired awareness seizures* (previously called *partial complex* or *petit mal seizures*) are often difficult to detect. Nonetheless, when present, they frequently interfere with the brain's ability to encode or store new memories. Such focal seizures should be considered when memory problems appear intermittently. The typical scenario is that you may notice fairly profound episodes of memory loss in a loved one, but when they undergo extensive memory testing as part of a neuropsychological evaluation, their memory is felt to be completely normal. If this occurs, obtaining an electroencephalogram (EEG) can be helpful.

Second, some individuals with chronic epilepsy may intermittently have prolonged seizures lasting more than a few minutes. If these prolonged seizures are difficult to stop, they are sometimes referred to as *status epilepticus*. Such prolonged seizures may damage the hippocampus permanently, leading to scarring of the hippocampus called *hippocampal sclerosis*. Not surprisingly, individuals with hippocampal sclerosis generally show impaired episodic memory.

Multiple Sclerosis

Multiple sclerosis is an autoimmune disease that affects patches of the white matter, the wiring of the brain. Because most of the brain's white matter is going to or from the frontal lobes, it is frontal lobe function that is most affected. This leads to difficulties similar to vascular cognitive impairment. Working memory capacity is diminished, and there is reduced ability to acquire new information and retrieve previously learned information from episodic memory. See the vascular cognitive impairment section of Chapter 13 for more information regarding the types of memory difficulties seen with damage to the white matter of the brain.

Strokes and Bleeds

Most strokes occur when an artery sending blood from the heart to the brain becomes blocked by a clot and a part of the brain doesn't receive enough blood and dies. There can also be bleeding strokes when a brain artery ruptures and blood suddenly accumulates inside the brain. Lastly, there are two types of bleeds between the brain and skull, called *subdural* and *epidural hematomas*. All of these strokes and bleeds can cause memory problems, usually due to one of three mechanisms.

First, the stroke or bleed may directly damage one of the memory centers, such as the hippocampus or its connections. Second, the stroke or bleed may put pressure on one of the memory centers or their connections. Third, an accumulation of strokes may cause vascular cognitive impairment or vascular dementia, as described in Chapter 13.

Strokes and bleeds can cause different types of memory problems depending upon where the damage occurs. If the stroke damages the hippocampus or its connections, episodic memory problems will usually be seen. If the damage occurs to the lower and outside part of the temporal lobe, then problems with semantic memory may be seen. And if the damage occurs to the basal ganglia or cerebellum, procedural memory problems are generally seen.

Strokes, whether clotting or bleeding, occur suddenly and are noticeable if large enough to cause memory problems. On the other hand, although subdural hematomas generally start after a fall, they may grow slowly over days or weeks and only then become large enough to cause memory problems.

The bottom line is that if you or a loved one experience memory loss suddenly or in the days or weeks after a fall, call the doctor immediately as a stroke or a bleed may have occurred.

Traumatic Brain Injury, Concussions, and Chronic Traumatic Encephalopathy

A traumatic brain injury occurs when there is an injury to the brain caused by an external force. When traumatic brain injuries are moderate or severe, many types of memory are affected, with the specifics depending upon which parts of the brain are injured. For example, injury to the cerebellum will affect procedural memory, whereas injury to the left temporal lobe will affect episodic and semantic memory.

A concussion is a mild traumatic brain injury that temporarily affects brain functioning. Memory loss around the time of injury is one of the most common symptoms of concussion, and the duration of amnesia has even been used as one of the criteria to define the severity of concussion. Individuals recovering from concussion frequently have difficulty concentrating, which affects their working memory, as well as their ability to acquire new information and retrieve previously learned information from episodic memory.

Individuals who have repetitive mild head impacts—not just two or three but hundreds or thousands, whether or not they meet criteria for concussion—are at risk for developing a progressive degenerative disease later in life known as chronic traumatic encephalopathy. Individuals who were boxers, American football players, or military veterans exposed to blast injuries are some of those who are at risk for chronic traumatic encephalopathy, as are those who have experienced intimate partner violence. Although this disease generally begins in microscopic regions of the frontal lobes, by the middle stage of the disease it spreads to the hippocampus. For this reason, individuals with chronic traumatic encephalopathy generally first experience trouble concentrating, affecting their working memory. As the disease progresses, their episodic memory abilities can be devastated, and they can end up with memory performance similar to that of individuals with Alzheimer's disease.

Transient Global Amnesia

Transient global amnesia is an unusual neurologic disorder in which individuals develop a sudden inability to form new memories along with the loss of a few hours or days of prior memories. They repeatedly ask questions like, "Where am I?" and "What's going on?" Approximately 5 minutes after giving the answers to them, they invariably repeat the same questions again. After ruling out other causes of sudden memory loss such as strokes, seizures, blood chemistry problems, and almost everything in this chapter, we are able to reassure the individual and their family that this type of memory loss is usually temporary and that their memory is likely to return within 24 hours (except for the time in which they could not form any new memories). Although no one is completely sure what causes transient global amnesia, it is more common in those with migraines and is often precipitated by the same things that trigger migraines.

PSYCHIATRIC DISORDERS

Here we will describe the memory problems that may be seen in some common psychiatric disorders, along with one psychiatric treatment, electroconvulsive therapy (ECT).

Anxiety

We've discussed anxiety and stress in several parts of this book (see Chapters 3, 7, and 9) because it can impair multiple types of memory in several different ways. First, when you're anxious or stressed, you may find yourself thinking about and preoccupied with whatever you are anxious or stressed about. These recurrent—and often intrusive—thoughts will diminish your ability to focus on what you want to, impairing your working memory capacity to keep information in mind and your episodic memory ability to learn new information and to retrieve previously learned information. Second, anxiety and stress cause hormones to be released into your bloodstream, such as adrenaline, that trigger your "fight or flight" response. This response forces your brain to pay attention to those things in your environment that could represent a threat—even if those things have absolutely nothing to do with your current goals. Again, your attention is diverted away from what you are trying to do with your working or episodic memory and is focused on what you are anxious about. High levels of the stress hormone cortisol can be detrimental to hippocampal function, making it harder to retrieve information from memory in the moment and, in cases of chronic stress and anxiety, relating to longer-lasting impairments in memory (see Chapter 15). Lastly, because information first needs to enter your episodic memory before it can become generalized, consolidated, and part of your long-term semantic memory, anxiety disrupts semantic memory as well—making it more difficult for you to learn that list of vocabulary words or biological pathways.

Depression

Like anxiety, depression can impair several types of memory in several different ways. If you're feeling sad, you may be preoccupied with thoughts about whatever is upsetting you. These sad thoughts may make it difficult for you to focus on what you're trying to learn or remember, impairing your ability to keep that desired information in your working memory, learn it with your episodic memory, or make it part of your semantic memory. Additionally, depression causes biological changes in the brain's chemistry and circuitry that can interfere with the proper function of the frontal lobes and the hippocampus—critical structures for working, episodic, and semantic memory.

Attention-Deficit/Hyperactivity Disorder (ADHD)

ADHD affects 8% to 12% of children worldwide,[5] making it the most common psychiatric disorder that affects memory. ADHD is a heterogeneous disorder with many different causes. Some researchers and clinicians believe that ADHD simply represents one end of a continuum of normal human behavior, with its symptomology perhaps a reflection of societal requirements for young children to sit still in a classroom for many hours each day. However, in certain cases it appears to be related to delayed maturity of the frontal lobes or their connections, and in others it may be related to a mild brain disorder affecting the frontal lobes, its connections, or related brain structures.

Whatever its cause and whether it is normal or abnormal, the majority of individuals who meet the diagnostic criteria for ADHD have diminished working memory compared to their age-matched peers. This diminished working memory leads to impaired ability to acquire new information with episodic memory, and therefore impaired ability to generalize and consolidate that new information into semantic memory. It is for this reason that children with ADHD have difficulty learning in school, as much of school involves acquiring new semantic information, such as vocabulary words, dates, facts, formulas, rules, and so forth.

Bipolar Disease

Formerly known as manic-depressive disorder, individuals with bipolar disease experience highly elevated happy moods that can rise into mania, as well as sad, depressed moods. We've already spoken about how depression can impair memory, and mania can impair memory as well. Although a happy, energetic mood often augments memory and productivity—perhaps enabling you to memorize your lines for your performance in the play in record time—when people are truly manic they have too much energy. They are overactive, cannot concentrate, and cannot focus on goal-directed activities. Thus, working, episodic, and semantic memory are all impaired.

Schizophrenia

In addition to other symptoms, individuals with schizophrenia experience hallucinations (typically hearing voices), delusions (such as paranoia), and disorganization in thinking and behavior. Not surprisingly, the majority of these individuals show impairments in working memory and thus episodic and semantic memory. The exact mechanism of these memory impairments is an active area of research. In fact, some researchers believe that understanding the nature of their memory impairment will also provide a better fundamental understanding of the disorder itself.

Nonetheless, there is a general consensus that some of the memory impairment stems from being distracted by internal stimuli—that is, it is hard to pay attention to what someone is saying to you if you are, at the same time, hearing voices in your head. And if your paranoia makes you think that everyone is deceiving you, you may be so preoccupied with trying to figure out how someone you just met is trying to trick you that you don't pay attention to their name.

In addition, research using functional magnetic resonance imaging (MRI) suggests that the brains of individuals with schizophrenia have abnormalities as well. Reduced activations are seen in the prefrontal cortex, hippocampus, and related structures in those with schizophrenia compared to healthy individuals.[6] Given the importance of the prefrontal cortex for working memory, both prefrontal cortex and hippocampus for episodic memory, and intact episodic memory for the creation of new semantic memories, it is not surprising that individuals with schizophrenia show impairment in working, episodic, and semantic memory.

Electroconvulsive Therapy

One highly effective treatment for severe depression that is not responsive to other therapies is ECT. The goal of this treatment is to cause a seizure (while using a medication to prevent convulsions of the body). ECT is typically given two or three times per week for a number of weeks. As mentioned earlier in this chapter, seizures cause memory loss. Although ECT, when properly performed, is not thought to cause permanent damage to the brain, impairment of autobiographical memory—the memories that make up our lives—is frequently observed. For example, Malin Blomberg, Åsa Hammar, and their colleagues in Bergen, Norway, evaluated memory performance in individuals with major depression who received ECT on the right hemisphere (the standard procedure). They found that although performance on standard neuropsychological tests of memory was unchanged by the ECT, ECT did impair retrieval of autobiographical memory 6 months after treatment.[7] Nonetheless, ECT works well in treating depression and several other disorders, so it still might be the best option for you or a loved one.

Dissociative Amnesia and Dissociative Identity Disorder

No discussion of memory loss due to psychiatric disorders would be complete without a discussion of the psychological disorders that can lead to amnesia. Although these are very real disorders—the individuals who have them are in no way "faking" their memory impairment—their cause is typically due to psychological trauma rather than to a known, direct change to brain structure or biochemistry as arises with amnesia brought about by brain injury or medication. Before going into more detail below, we feel obliged to mention that the typical movie involving either of these two conditions is often not consistent with the medically observed disorders.

In *dissociative amnesia* (a disorder that now subsumes the older terms *psychogenic amnesia* and *dissociative fugue*), individuals experience an inability to recall important personal information that would not typically be lost with ordinary forgetting as we describe in Chapter 8. Prior to diagnosis, brain problems such as strokes, seizures, and transient global amnesia must be ruled out. Once these and other neurologic causes are eliminated, the most common cause is an experienced or witnessed traumatic event, such as physical or sexual abuse, rape, combat, genocide, natural disasters, or death of a loved one. Other causes include significant internal conflict, such as tremendous guilt or remorse after criminal behavior, or seemingly unresolvable interpersonal difficulties. Usually the amnesia is localized or selective, confined to the inability to recall specific events or a series of events. For example, the individual may not recall days fighting in intense combat, or minutes witnessing a horrific event. More rarely the amnesia is generalized, such that the individual cannot recall their identity and life history. In addition to forgetting events, those with generalized amnesia may also lose access to well-learned skills and knowledge, thus showing problems in episodic, procedural, and semantic memory. Unlike with other causes of amnesia, most cases of dissociative amnesia resolve relatively quickly (often within days), with the memories becoming accessible again.

In *dissociative identity disorder* (previously called *multiple personality disorder*), individuals have two or more personality states. It generally develops in childhood due to prolonged and severe physical, sexual, and/or emotional abuse. Memories that were formed in one identity may or may not be accessible by another identity, such that from the perspective of the individual, their family, and their doctors there may be gaps in memory that are apparently unexplainable. Different than dissociative amnesia, in dissociative identity disorder the forgotten times and events may be ordinary and nontraumatic.

Alcohol and Drugs

What about use—or abuse—of alcohol and drugs? These are such important causes of memory loss that we devote an entire chapter to them (Chapter 19).

THERE ARE MANY CAUSES OF MEMORY LOSS

So, did you figure out the problem with our 32-year-old man discussed at the beginning of the chapter? Do you see that it doesn't quite fit with dissociative amnesia, despite occurring in the setting of sexual activity? After considering all of the conditions listed below, this man was most likely experiencing transient global amnesia, a benign condition associated with migraines, as described earlier in this chapter.

- Medication side effects (especially anticholinergics, antihistamines, typical antipsychotics, and benzodiazepines)
- Vitamin deficiencies (especially vitamin B_{12}, B_1, and D)
- Hormonal imbalances (including thyroid disorders)
- Bodily stress, infections, and diseases (including Lyme disease, COVID-19, encephalitis, diabetes, major surgeries and anesthesia, organ failure, and poor sleep)
- Neurologic disorders (including brain tumors, epilepsy and seizures, multiple sclerosis, strokes, transient global amnesia, and traumatic brain injury)

- Psychiatric disorders (including anxiety, depression, ADHD, bipolar disease, schizophrenia, ECT, dissociative amnesia, and alcohol or drug use)

* * *

After considering common disorders that can cause you to forget, we're ready to consider disorders that prevent you from forgetting normally, such as post-traumatic stress disorder.

15

Post-traumatic stress disorder

When you can't forget

In 2001, psychologist Margaret McKinnon sat next to her husband on an Air Transat overnight flight from Toronto to Lisbon, Portugal. The newlyweds were midway over the Atlantic when the flurry of announcements began. The pilot was having difficulty. Passengers should outfit themselves with life vests and prepare for a "ditching" in the ocean. For 30 minutes, passengers waited as the plane's systems failed one after another and the aircraft lurched, jostling them and their belongings. People screamed. Prayed. Some fainted. And then, at the last moment, land—and then a runway—came into sight. The pilot had located a small island in the Azores with a military base. Amidst the screamed instructions to "brace, brace, brace," the plane glided to a successful landing. Everyone survived, most without serious physical injuries.

This is a true story, with about the happiest ending anyone could have imagined. But, over time, it became clear that it was not just an ending. It was also the opening chapter to a story that would unfold differently for different passengers. Over time, some passengers felt they had moved on from the harrowing experience, leaving it in their past. Others continued to re-experience the event—in their thoughts, memories, and nightmares—even as they adjusted their behavior so as to avoid reminders of it: all quintessential symptoms of post-traumatic stress disorder, better known by its initials, PTSD.

In this chapter, we examine what happens to memory for individuals experiencing PTSD, for whom today's experiences are disrupted by the echo of yesterday's trauma.

THE MEMORY SCAR

In *Principles of Psychology* in 1890, the psychologist and philosopher William James wrote, "An impression may be so exciting emotionally as almost to leave a scar on the cerebral tissues." "Scar" is an apt word choice. It conjures the damage that a traumatic event can bring into people's futures. It more generally envisages the seeming permanence of an emotional memory, the sense that the event is seared into our minds forever. There is a shallower forgetting curve for emotional memories than for more mundane experiences. And while we lose or distort some of the details of emotional memories, just as we do for memories of mundane experiences, we are likely to retain at least the gist of what happened.

MEMORIES OF TRAUMA

Dr. McKinnon, as a psychological scientist, soon realized the Air Transat flight provided an unparalleled opportunity to examine memory for a traumatic event, and to compare the memory patterns for those who were and were not experiencing PTSD. The onboard experiences were well documented: There were records of when announcements were made, when cabin lights went off, and when oxygen masks deployed. Everyone on that plane had experienced those events in exactly the same sequence. But how would the details of the event be remembered by individual passengers?

She and her colleagues discovered that, even several years later, passengers remembered many details of the event vividly—many more than from other events around that same time period. When they looked at patterns of brain activity in a small group of passengers, they found that the amygdala—that tiny, almond-shaped brain structure involved with emotions—was robustly engaged during the retrieval of these negative memories, in concert with regions typically observed in episodic memory retrieval.[1]

CONTROLLING THE NARRATIVE

This ability to vividly remember the event details did not distinguish individuals who were experiencing PTSD from those who were not, nor did the accuracy of the memories. But there were some intriguingly different memory patterns. When Dr. McKinnon asked the survivors to describe what happened on the flight, those who had developed PTSD provided more commentary on the event and facts about its occurrence, and they also had more repetitions in their episodic recalls than did those not experiencing PTSD. It was as if those with PTSD could not rein in their memory, providing extraneous facts and commentary rather than narrowing onto the more direct experience of the flight.

The very features that made this event well suited to study memory for trauma also made it hard to know whether these findings would generalize to other forms of trauma. The passengers experienced a single traumatic event, with the threat of death lasting for many minutes; they experienced it collectively, often with a loved one seated nearby; and the researchers only studied adults. Dr. McKinnon and her colleagues acknowledged that memory patterns may differ for repeated traumas,

for traumas experienced in childhood, or for single-event traumas of a different duration or experienced in different social
contexts.

Despite these caveats, the results seen in these passengers
do—at least in a broad sense—align with other research suggesting that PTSD may rob individuals of their control over memory retrieval. Sometimes, this disrupted control seems to result
in a fragmented memory: one that is disorganized or is missing
details from the worst moments of the trauma. The individual
may still be able to give a general account of what happened—
perhaps relying on a narrative that they have rehearsed—but
they lack control over the way they re-experience the traumatic
event.[2]

AN INTRUSIVE MEMORY

With less control over their re-experience, individuals with
PTSD often find themselves experiencing intrusive memories
of the trauma. Intrusive memories describe those that spring
to mind involuntarily—often with rich sensory-perceptual
features—in ways that are disruptive to daily functioning. An
individual may re-experience portions of the sights or sounds
or smells associated with a traumatic event, jolting them from
the present into a moment of past trauma.

Intrusive memories are not unique to those with PTSD; they
co-occur across many psychiatric disorders,[3] and may even be
a common reaction to a traumatic event. For instance, in one
study of individuals who had been in a motor vehicle accident,
approximately 75% of people reported having intrusive memories in the first few weeks following the accident.[4] With the
majority of individuals experiencing or witnessing a traumatic
event in their lifetime,[5] this means that most of us are likely to
at some point have the experience of an intrusive memory.

In the moments immediately following a trauma, the involuntary retrieval of the experience may even be adaptive. Dorthe

Berntsen at Aarhus University in Denmark has suggested that there could be initial benefits to being reminded of the trauma. Those reminders might help to prevent re-exposure to the danger. But, over time, their benefits are likely to dissipate, and therefore in the usual case, the involuntary memories should subside.[6]

Indeed, with distance from the traumatic event, intrusive memories do typically dissipate. By 3 months after a motor vehicle accident, only 25% of individuals still reported intrusive memories.[4] But in those with PTSD, the intrusive memories persist, and their presence is a core clinical feature of the disorder.

WHEN FORGETTING FAILS

As discussed in Chapter 11, people can—with effort— put information out of mind so that it does not return at unwanted moments. Michael Anderson and colleagues analogize it to how we can suppress a muscle action: Our instinct might be to reach for an object falling off of a kitchen counter, but if that object is a knife, we try to suppress the reaching action and let the knife fall. In the same way, when we are cued by reminders of an event that we would prefer not to remember, we can attempt to suppress the retrieval process.[7] These attempts can, over time, reduce the accessibility of the memories,[8] allowing us to avoid the metaphorical scar of the memory just as we could avoid the physical scar from the knife.

But for individuals with PTSD, attempts to forget are often futile. Individuals with PTSD struggle to put information out of mind, even when they are told it is irrelevant or should be suppressed.[7,9] Interestingly, this inability to keep memories out of mind relates to the severity of PTSD symptoms—the greater the inability to suppress memories, the more severe the PTSD symptoms. Though intrusive memories are a key symptom of

PTSD, an intriguing possibility is that PTSD may be as much a disorder of forgetting as it is a disorder of remembering.

FLASHBACKS OF COMBAT

Although the terminology of PTSD came into prominence around 1980, in the aftermath of the Vietnam conflict, the psychological stress of war has been recognized since ancient times. The Greek historian Herodotus noted something akin to PTSD when describing a combat survivor in the Battle of Marathon in 490 BC, and the psychological effects of combat were labeled as "Da Costa's syndrome" during the Civil War, "shell shock" during World War I, and "battle fatigue" during World War II.[10] Over time, we have come to understand that the symptoms of PTSD are not a result of artillery bursts physically damaging the nervous system (literally, "shell shock") but rather a result of the emotional trauma of combat. (Note, however, that in some cases blast injuries may also cause damage to the nervous system leading to blast-related traumatic brain injury or eventually to chronic traumatic encephalopathy, as discussed in Chapter 14.)

Indeed, the severe stress experienced during combat is powerful in its ability to elicit PTSD. At any given time, about 10% to 15% of combat-exposed veterans are currently diagnosed with PTSD, and approximately one-third of combat-exposed veterans will at some point in their life meet the diagnostic criteria for PTSD.[11] These individuals, like others with PTSD, often suffer "flashbacks" and re-experience fragments of their traumatic event in harrowing sensory detail. They may hear a weapon's discharge, smell burning rubber, or taste dust as they inhale. These sensations can catapult them to the moment of their past trauma.

Disturbed Sleep

For many with PTSD, sleep provides no reprieve, their nights filled with vivid, recurring nightmares.[12] These nightmares may be the result of the brain's bombardment by sensory activity even while asleep. Sleep patterns are altered in combat veterans with PTSD, and some of the disruptions suggest that the sleeping brain fails to effectively gate the flow of sensory information.[13] This failure may lead to the sensory-intense nightmares while asleep and, with sleep not serving its typical role of stripping the emotional intensity and sensory details away from a memory (see Chapter 20), may also contribute to the flashbacks experienced during the waking day.

Shrinking from Stress

Given the critical role of the hippocampus in memory, it may come as no surprise that alterations to this region's structure and function are implicated in PTSD. For instance, one study that examined multiple brain structures in over 1,800 individuals with or without PTSD found significantly smaller hippocampal volumes in individuals with PTSD.[14]

These findings may reflect reductions in hippocampal volume as a result of the experienced stressor. The experience of severe stress, such as occurs in combat, can trigger a cascade of processes, resulting in the release of very high levels of neurochemicals that may be disruptive to cell growth and function—especially in the hippocampus. Alternatively, it may be that having a larger hippocampus at the time of severe stress exposure may protect individuals from developing PTSD. In studies that enroll identical twins, not only do combat veterans without PTSD tend to show larger hippocampi than combat veterans with PTSD, the same patterns are also revealed in their identical twins who have never served in combat.[15]

IS PTSD A MEMORY DISORDER?

PTSD is categorized as an anxiety disorder but, over the past decade, scientists have questioned whether it would be more apt to characterize it as a memory disorder. Certainly, memory disturbances are prominent in PTSD, and are required for diagnostic criteria to be met. But are those memory disturbances merely a symptom of PTSD—or might they be an underlying cause?

Some models of PTSD suggest that intrusive memories may drive the other symptoms.[16,17] Avoidance behaviors may stem from people's desire to minimize exposure to cues that trigger the memories. The unwanted memories may lead to the negative alterations in cognition and mood: It's hard to focus on other tasks at hand and to effectively regulate emotions while being bombarded with unpleasant memories at inopportune times.

The "mnemonic model" of PTSD put forth by David Rubin and his colleagues at Duke University puts memory even more squarely in the crosshairs of PTSD treatment.[18] Traditionally, there has been extensive focus on what *event features* may relate to the prevalence of developing PTSD or the nature of the symptoms experienced in PTSD. The mnemonic model emphasizes that, with events such as the Air Transat flight as a rare exception, clinicians have little traction into the actual traumatic event that a person experienced. Instead, clinicians are treating a person's response to their memory for the traumatic event, a memory that—as we discussed throughout Part 2—can be influenced by a variety of factors. Thus, the therapeutic target in PTSD is the memory representation itself.

On the one hand, a memory-centric model of PTSD is necessarily simplified. PTSD is a complex disorder that can affect many facets of a person's cognitive functioning, emotional well-being, and social integration. On the other hand, treatments that focus on treating the memory characteristics—reducing the intensity or frequency of the intrusive memories using behavioral therapy or, potentially, medications such as prazosin—are often effective in restoring other domains of functioning.[2] As we understand more about the malleability of memory and gain tools to disrupt memory's storage and retrieval mechanisms, considering PTSD a disorder of memory may suggest new treatments to improve the day-to-day experience of trauma survivors. Although we do not know exactly what such new treatments might look like, we will return to this topic of how the brain deals with emotional trauma in Chapter 20, when we discuss sleep.

MEMORY IS ALTERED IN PTSD

- Individuals with PTSD often re-experience memories of their trauma. The memories feel intrusive, and they persist long after the event.
- Individuals with PTSD often report global difficulties with concentration or with committing new information to memory.
- PTSD is associated with a disruption in sleep, which may further exacerbate the memory challenges.
- Although memory disturbances have long been recognized as a prominent feature of PTSD, ongoing research is examining whether the way that memory structures are built and reassembled over time may play a more direct and causal role in PTSD.

16

Those who remember everything

Whenever I see a date flash on the television (or anywhere else, for that matter) I automatically go back to that day and remember where I was, what I was doing, what day it fell on and on and on and on and on. It is non-stop, uncontrollable.—Jill Price

What happened on the 10th of March, 1983? What day of the week was August 8, 2008? What was the weather like on January 31, 2021? Unless we happened to choose a date with special significance to you, perhaps a birthday or anniversary, you most likely have no idea what the answer to these questions is. But for a small group of people—such as Jill Price, as quoted by the neurobiologist and memory researcher Jim McGaugh[1]— answering these questions is nearly as easy as answering what they ate for breakfast this morning. Sure, it may take a moment to retrieve the content, but the details are there, waiting to be brought to mind.

In this chapter, we'll explore individuals who have an extraordinary ability to remember—whether they try to or not.

THE MYTH OF PHOTOGRAPHIC MEMORY

We first want to dismiss a common misconception, which is that there are people with "photographic memory," or the ability to briefly look at something—a page of a book, or a photograph—and recall all of its details accurately for a long period of time. There is no scientific evidence for the existence of this ability. The memory phenomenon that comes closest is *eidetic memory*,[2] which describes a visual after-image of sorts that allows individuals to hold details in mind for seconds or minutes—long enough to recount them, but still a quickly-fading representation. Unlike the concept of photographic memory, eidetic memory does not lead to a picture-perfect recounting of details; just as with all of our memories, eidetic memories lack some details and can assume details that were not really there. Eidetic memory is somewhat common in children[3] but occurs incredibly rarely in adults, leading some to hypothesize that this visual ability may be disrupted by the development of language.

EXPERTISE AND MEMORY

When adults show an ability to remember large quantities of information in great detail, it usually is linked either to the engagement of specific memory strategies (see Part 5) or to domains of expertise. As mentioned in Chapter 8, when highly ranked chess players were briefly shown a chessboard with pieces arranged in a logical way, the player could look away and recreate the board from memory with near-perfect accuracy every time. But, if that same player was shown a board with pieces arranged randomly, their memory suffered.[4] There was nothing particularly remarkable about the chess player's *memory*, but there was something remarkable about their chess *expertise*; their knowledge of the game provided them with powerful organizing principles to help them group distinct chess pieces into sets, reducing the memory demands.

SELF-EXPERTISE

Fortunately, even if you haven't gained expertise in any specialized domains like chess, you have developed expertise in at least one thing: yourself! People orient automatically upon hearing their name, and naturally think about how information in the world relates to them. You can use that expertise to help you remember information that you consider relevant to yourself. Extensive research shows that you will better remember information that you're asked to process in relation to yourself rather than in relation to another person.[5]

Let's try a little experiment. Think about whether you'd answer each of these questions in the affirmative or the negative:

Are you honest? Is your neighbor serious? Are you reliable? Are you quiet? Is your neighbor ambitious? Is your neighbor outgoing? Are you respectful? Are you wise? Is your neighbor witty? Are you patient? Is your neighbor loyal? Is your neighbor kind? Are you hopeful?

Now, try to recall all of the adjectives that appeared in these questions. Typically, individuals do better remembering the adjectives they've been asked to think about in relation to themselves (in this example, honest, reliable, quiet, respectful, wise, patient, and hopeful) than those they've been asked to think about in relation to another person.

REMEMBERING EVERY YESTERDAY

For a small group of individuals, they don't just show a slight benefit in the ability to remember information that is relevant to them; they remember nearly every moment from their past.

It is an ability termed *highly superior autobiographical memory.*[1]
Autobiographical is an important part of this term, qualifying
that the superior memory does not extend to all domains. Most
of these individuals show variable performance on laboratory
assessments of memory; some are good at remembering numbers or faces, others not so much. Many forget where they put
their glasses. They do not show anything that approximates the
mythic "photographic memory." But when it comes to remembering how their past has unfolded, their memories work in
ways that are fascinatingly different from the way that most of
us remember: It is as if they can rewind to certain dates and re-
experience events with astonishing clarity.

There seems little doubt that there is something qualitatively
different about these individuals' memories. If these individuals were simply at the extreme of a continuum of memory
ability, we would expect to find many individuals who fall else-
where along the continuum. We would expect there to be those
who might not remember nearly every day from their past, but
who still remember far more past days than most of us—those
who might have *superior* but not *highly superior* autobiographical memory. So far, there has not been strong evidence for this
gradation[1]; it seems as though these individuals may be members of a select group, able to accomplish feats of memory that
most of us cannot achieve. That, of course, doesn't mean we
cannot get closer to these individuals' abilities, with hard work
and engagement of effective strategies, such as those described
in Part 5.

Even for these individuals, the general principles of memory
that we described in Part 2 still mostly seem to apply. Their
memories aren't perfect. They, too, forget some details of past
events. And, like the rest of us, their memories can be susceptible
to misinformation. In one study, experimenters provided misinformation about a video of a plane crash (no video existed).[6]
A number of participants—even those with *highly superior*

autobiographical memory—later falsely remembered seeing the video. But while some general principles of memory—like its reconstructive nature—seem to persist, there is no question of these individuals' extraordinary memory abilities, with only about 100 such individuals being identified worldwide.[1]

CALENDAR SAVANTS

Some individuals with developmental disorders or other causes of brain injury show extraordinary abilities in a particular area despite significant impairments in many mental domains. These individuals are referred to as *savants*. Savants are most commonly those with autism, a neurodevelopmental spectrum disorder characterized by social and communicative impairments along with repetitive behaviors and restricted interests. While some savants show remarkable talents in music, drawing, or calculation, many are *calendar savants*. These individuals are able to determine the day of the week for dates that fall within a large time range, and many can also solve the reverse problem, providing the date for a particular day of the month (e.g., What was the date of the third Wednesday in April 1987?)

Memory and Mental Math

It is poorly understood how calendar savants solve these problems. Many calendar savants show deep interest in the Gregorian calendar system and will spend hours studying it. It is likely that they can then use a combination of memory and relatively simple calculations, based on calendar regularities, to arrive at the answers. We all know that there are seven days to the week and can therefore quickly make some deductions about day–date pairings (e.g., the 1st, 8th, 15th, 22nd, and 29th of the month must always be the same day of the week). But there are many other regularities that can be capitalized upon. For example: April and July always have the same starting day; in non-leap years, January and

October also have matched starting days, as do February, March, and November. With very few exceptions, the day–date calendar structure repeats itself exactly every 28 years. This knowledge can be used to solve date problems. Some savants may also rely on memory for specific day–date pairings (e.g., March 3, 2019, was a Sunday), using basic week-and-month patterns to determine surrounding day–date couplings.

Calendars on the Brain

Case studies that have examined the brain activity while calendar savants solve date problems have provided evidence consistent with the use of memory strategies as well as mental computations. One savant, asked to associate a day of the week with the corresponding calendar date, showed activation in the hippocampus, temporal lobe, and frontal lobe—all regions consistent with long-term memory.[7] Another savant, asked to indicate whether a day–date match was true or false, showed increased activity in regions of the parietal lobe associated with working memory and mental calculations, and these regions were engaged more when more remote dates were queried.[8]

Mental Calendars Versus Mental Diaries

While working memory and long-term episodic and semantic memory may be used to solve date problems, outstanding autobiographical memory is not required for calendar savantism. The memory feats of calendar savants are quite different than the memory feats of those with highly superior autobiographical memory. While many of us might solve date problems by relying on our autobiographical memories, this does not appear to be how calendar savants solve these problems (see Figure 16.1). In fact, one calendar savant, age 25, presented with severely impaired episodic memory, performing below the first percentile on many tasks of episodic memory, and was classified as showing "definitely abnormal" performance for autobiographical experiences.[9] Yet some calendar savants do also show

Question: What day of the week was Dec. 18th, 1980?

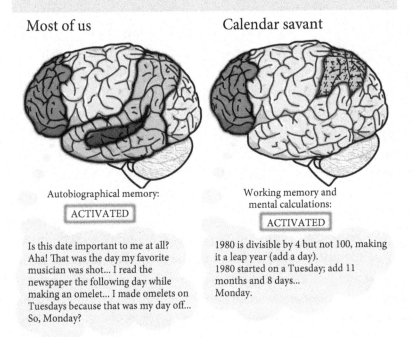

Most of us   Calendar savant

Autobiographical memory: Working memory and
                                          mental calculations:

ACTIVATED   ACTIVATED

Is this date important to me at all?   1980 is divisible by 4 but not 100, making
Aha! That was the day my favorite   it a leap year (add a day).
musician was shot... I read the   1980 started on a Tuesday; add 11
newspaper the following day while   months and 8 days...
making an omelet... I made omelets on   Monday.
Tuesdays because that was my day off...
So, Monday?

Figure 16.1. Many calendar savants solve date problems differently than the rest of us.

highly accurate memory for past personal events. In one study, a parent provided receipts that documented specific events that had occurred over a 7-year time period. When the savant, age 15, was given the date on the receipt, he was remarkably accurate at recalling the event that the receipt corroborated, despite the fact that many of these experiences were fairly mundane events, such as a family dinner at a restaurant.[10]

THE BRAINS OF EXTRAORDINARY REMEMBERERS

You might expect that the brains of extraordinary rememberers would look quite different than the brains of typical remembers. But, so far, the differences revealed have been subtle, without any apparent anatomical differences by visual inspection. Although there are a number of differences in brain structure and connectivity when comparing those with autism to typically developing peers,[11] it is not yet clear if there are systematic differences between the brains of autistic savants and autistic individuals without savant abilities.

When peering into the brains of individuals with highly superior autobiographical memory using magnetic resonance imaging (MRI) methods, a few possible differences have been noted. In one individual, there was increased volume in the right amygdala, and evidence of increased functional connectivity between the amygdala and hippocampus.[12] These results make sense given the critical role of the hippocampus in episodic memory, and the ability of the amygdala to increase the efficacy of hippocampal function. Looking at a small group of individuals who performed extremely well on a test of personal autobiographical memory,[13] there were increases in the gray matter of the parahippocampal gyrus (as the name suggests, this is the tissue surrounding the hippocampus), and also evidence that a particular white-matter pathway that speeds communication between the frontal lobe and temporal lobe (the lobe containing the parahippocampal gyrus) was particularly robust in the high performers. Taken together, these results may suggest that highly superior autobiographical memory is made possible by relatively subtle changes in the structure of circuitry critical for typical episodic remembering.

BECOMING A BETTER REMEMBERER

It's important to keep in mind that remembering *every* detail or *every* daily experience is rarely a necessary or even useful goal; as described in Part 2, culling some of the details can be helpful for seeing the connections between experiences and for efficient decision-making. But nevertheless, there are important lessons we can learn from those with extraordinary memory. While it can be easy to lament all the ways in which we are different from those with extraordinary memory, in some important ways, they are capitalizing on two broad capacities that all of us can benefit from:

- **Gain expertise.** Just like the chess players, or the calendar savants who came to their knowledge through hours spent analyzing the calendar system, we all can work to gain expertise in specific domains and use that expertise to enable better remembering.
- **Be present.** In her book *Total Memory Makeover*,[14] Marilu Henner (from the television sitcom *Taxi*), one of the approximately 100 individuals with highly superior autobiographical memory, has this to say: "When we participate actively in our lives and open our senses to all the stimuli around us, we build memories that can be retrieved and enjoyed the rest of our lives." Her point is an excellent one. We all can remember better by staying in the present moment, and by embracing the information coming through our senses rather than distracting ourselves with our phones or mental to-do lists.

To learn more about how to achieve better memory and capitalize upon the advice of Marilu Henner, we invite you to continue with Part 4: Do the right things and Part 5: Techniques to remember better.

Part 4

DO THE RIGHT THINGS

17

Exercise

The elixir of life

What if we told you that there was a magical potion you could drink daily to help you sleep, lift your mood, and—most importantly—improve your memory? What if we also told you that this same potion could make your body physiologically younger—literally extending your life? Perhaps this potion bubbled out of an enchanted spring located at the top of a hill that you had to climb 30 minutes each day to reach. Would you climb the hill to gain such a miraculous elixir of life, youth, sleep, happiness, and memory? Of course you would. Now, let's say that you've been climbing this hill and drinking from the spring daily over the last year. You've confirmed the potion's miraculous effects: You've become stronger, healthier, and more physically fit. You feel good, sleep soundly each night, and can remember information better. One day, as you reach the top of the hill, we are there waiting for you. We explain that the spring you are drinking from contains only pure water, and that what has wrought the magical changes to your body, sleep, mood, and memory is the journey you take each day up and down the hill. We go on to tell you that, in fact, any such moderately strenuous 30-minute daily journey will allow you to continue to reap the same benefits. Wouldn't you be overjoyed to hear this news?

We hope that you would be overjoyed, because it's actually all true—every word of it. Exercise really is the elixir of life, youth, sleep, happiness, and memory. We don't mean to say that it makes any of those things perfect, but it really does make you physiologically younger, extend your life, help you sleep, lift your mood, and improve your memory. That's why we've chosen to start with exercise in reviewing the things that you can do to help you remember better. We'll now discuss how much exercise to do, what type of exercise to do, and some of the data revealing the benefits of exercise. But first, a word of caution.

CHECK WITH YOUR DOCTOR

It is important to check with your doctor prior to starting a completely new exercise program. Checking with your doctor is especially critical if you have a family history of heart disease, are a current or former smoker, are overweight, or have any of the following conditions: high cholesterol, high blood pressure, diabetes or prediabetes (high blood sugar levels), asthma or other lung disease, arthritis, or kidney disease. Lastly, if you experience any of the following warning signs when you are exercising you should seek immediate medical attention by calling your doctor or dialing 911 (in most regions of the United States): pain or discomfort in your chest, neck, jaw, arms, or legs; dizziness or fainting; shortness of breath; ankle swelling; rapid heartbeat; leg pain; or other symptoms you are concerned about.

You also want to speak with your doctor about which exercises would be best for you if you have any joint pains or other orthopedic or medical conditions. For example, swimming may be better than jogging if you have knee or hip problems. And there are vigorous arm exercise machines available for those who cannot use their legs.

IT'S NEVER TOO LATE TO START EXERCISING—OR TOO EARLY

Wondering if you're too old to start exercising? Studies have shown that even older individuals in their 70s, 80s, and 90s benefit from participating in regular exercise.[1] Other studies show that beginning a vigorous exercise program in midlife can delay the onset of dementia by almost 10 years.[2] So, whether you are 29 or 92, it is a great age to start exercising.

WHAT TYPE AND HOW MUCH EXERCISE SHOULD YOU DO?

Aerobic Exercise

Recommendations from organizations such as the Centers for Disease Control, the American Congress of Sports Medicine, and the National Institutes of Health agree that the *minimum* recommended amount of exercise is 30 minutes of moderate aerobic activity, 5 days each week. Aerobic exercise is any activity that gets your heart beating faster and your lungs breathing harder. A brisk walk for 30 minutes is an example of a moderate aerobic activity, whereas a jog covering more distance for the same amount of time would be a more strenuous activity. If your heart, lungs, bones, joints, and other parts of your body are healthy and strong, doing more vigorous exercise for 60 minutes daily would be better for your brain health.

Other good examples of aerobic exercise are swimming, cycling, rowing, as well as using an elliptical trainer or an upper body (arm only) ergometer. You can take aerobics, Zumba, dance, or spin classes. You can also participate in sports such as basketball, tennis, soccer, hockey, skiing, and golf (if you walk rather than ride in the cart). Not sure what is the best exercise for you? Try out different ones and see which you like best. One of the most important aspects of the exercise you do is that you enjoy it enough to do it most if not every day. Cross-training—doing different exercises on different days—is a good way to reduce the wear and tear on your bones and joints and will also allow you to strengthen different muscles in addition to getting your heart pumping hard.

Exercise for Strength, Balance, and Flexibility

Also recommended are at least 2 hours each week of activities that help with strength, balance, and flexibility, such as yoga, tai chi, and Pilates. In addition to being good for the health of your body, these types of exercises are important for brain health because they help to prevent falls—a major cause of head injury. Falls increase with age, such that one of every three adults over age 65 falls each year. About one-quarter of those who fall suffer a serious consequence such as a head injury, which can lead to permanent cognitive impairment or even death.

REDUCE YOUR RISK OF STROKE

Strokes are a major cause of impairment in memory and thinking. A sedentary lifestyle is one of the major risk factors for the development of strokes. Exercise can help to minimize many of the conditions that are risk factors for strokes. Exercise helps promote weight loss, which can reduce the risk of stroke for those who are overweight or obese. Compared to those adults who maintain a healthy weight, overweight adults are 22% more likely to suffer a stroke and obese adults are 64% more likely.[3] This increase in risk was even greater for young adults, who had a 36% and 81% increase in stroke risk from being overweight and obese, respectively.[4] Exercise reduces the levels of "bad" low-density lipoproteins (LDL) cholesterol while increasing the levels of "good" high-density lipoproteins (HDL). Exercise lowers your blood pressure and your risk of diabetes. And even those with diabetes have better control over their blood sugars if they exercise. For all these reasons, exercise reduces the risk of strokes.

SLEEP WELL

As we will discuss in detail in Chapter 20, sleep is critical for proper memory function. Whether you are young or old, exercise helps you to sleep better. Those who exercise regularly report better quality of sleep as well as a reduction in the time it takes to fall asleep and the number of times they wake up in the night. They also report less need for medications—important since there are almost no medications for sleep that don't impair memory (the exception being melatonin; see Chapter 20). Exercise at a time that is convenient for you and that you can work into your daily routine. Just remember that exercise can actually keep you awake if you do it right before bed, and it may take a few months of regular exercise to get the maximal sleep-boosting effect.

FEEL GOOD

We discussed in Chapter 14 how anxiety and depression can impair your memory and thinking. Luckily, exercise reduces anxiety and depression. Exercise can also brighten your mood even if you don't have anxiety or depression. You may experience this mood-boosting effect within minutes of engaging in exercise, but you will also find that its effects generally persist over the next 24 hours. Exercise increases your brain's levels of serotonin and norepinephrine—the chemicals that lift your mood. That exercise increases these chemicals also teaches your body how to deal more effectively with physical and psychological stress. Exercise can sometimes produce a sense of euphoria—the runner's high—due to the release of endocannabinoids (chemicals our body makes that are similar to some of those found in cannabis).[5] Exercise can also help you socialize more if you join an exercise class or a gym or you go out for a walk outside. Exercise can give you a sense of accomplishment. For all these reasons, not only can exercise reduce your anxiety and depression but it can also do it almost as effectively as medications—and with fewer side effects.[6]

BULK UP YOUR BRAIN

The most exciting thing to tell you about exercise and memory is that exercise releases growth factors in the brain that can actually enlarge the size of your hippocampus and improve your memory. These effects, seen in young, middle-aged, and older adults, can be observed as quickly as 6 weeks and are persistent—with continued exercise—for at least a year.[7,8] The increase in hippocampal volume is about 2%, which is equivalent to reversing age-related shrinkage by 1 to 2 years. Exercise increases the level of a chemical called *brain-derived neurotrophic factor (BDNF)*, and one study found that the amount of this factor that was released correlated with the increase in hippocampal volume, and that correlated with the improvement in memory performance.[8]

How does BDNF work its magic to increase hippocampal volume and memory performance? Most researchers believe BDNF works by increasing the number of new brain cells formed in the hippocampus, either by promoting their development or by protecting their survival.[9] That sentence may or may not be surprising to you, but it was initially surprising to us, because when we were in school, the dogma was that adult humans didn't make any new brain cells. But we now know that you do—all throughout your life. And guess what part of your brain makes more new cells than any other? Yes, that's right, your hippocampus. The bottom line is that when you exercise, you release growth factors in your brain that grow new brain cells and improve your memory performance.

EXERCISE FOR MENTAL FLEXIBILITY

Have you ever felt particularly mentally sharp after a vigorous hike in which you navigated your way along a series of paths? If so, you've witnessed first-hand that exercise can help your working memory, the ability to flexibly juggle information in mind (see Chapter 3). These benefits can be seen during and immediately after exercising.[10] Some of these benefits may be particularly large when exercise includes both an aerobic component (as you climb the hill) and a cognitive component (as you navigate the hiking trails).

EXERCISE, ALZHEIMER'S DISEASE, AND DEMENTIA

Exercise can reduce your risk of developing Alzheimer's disease and related dementias. One study looked at the size of the hippocampus in individuals with the *APOE-e4* gene that increases the risk of Alzheimer's disease before and after starting an exercise program. After a year and a half, those who were sedentary experienced a 3% shrinkage while those who exercised consistently had virtually none.[11] And, as we mentioned earlier, a vigorous exercise program in midlife can delay the onset of dementia by almost 10 years.[2]

Even those already diagnosed with Alzheimer's disease in the mild cognitive impairment or mild dementia stages can benefit from exercise, with some studies showing improvement in memory and thinking and others showing preserved function and improved quality of life.[12,13]

MAKE AN EXERCISE PLAN

So, what are you waiting for? Make a plan to fit at least 30 minutes of exercise, 5 days each week, into your life. Remember that adding a little bit more vigorous exercise, increasing to 60 minutes duration, and exercising daily will all produce greater benefits, so long as it is healthy for your body (see the *Check with Your Doctor* section earlier in this chapter). Begin with small, specific goals that you can accomplish and build up from there. Build in contingency plans for bad weather. For example, "I'm going to walk briskly 5 days this week for 30 minutes each day either outside enjoying the scenery or inside listening to music." Make your commitment to exercise lifelong. Climb up that hill and start drinking the elixir of life: exercise.

EXERCISE FOR OPTIMAL MEMORY

Keep your mind strong by keeping your body fit.

- Check in with your doctor prior to starting a brand-new exercise program, if you're not sure what the best exercise is for you, or if you're experiencing any discomfort while exercising.
- Perform aerobic exercise 5 to 7 days each week for 30 to 60 minutes each day.
- Exercise for strength, balance, and flexibility at least 2 hours each week.

18

Nutrition

You are what you eat

You open your refrigerator and reach for the 2-liter bottle of diet cola, lean beef patties, and low-fat hot dogs. Moving to the cupboard, you pull down the reduced-calorie white bread rolls for the burgers and dogs, and the extra-slim potato chips. After dinner, you have some reduced-fat cream-filled cookies. You grimace slightly as you pat your upset stomach, thinking, "Well, the advertisements say these foods are supposed to be healthy, but they don't make me feel very good!"

"You are what you eat" is an old saying that has a lot of truth to it. The foods you consume are used to build the amino acids, proteins, lipids, nucleic acids, and other molecules that make up your body and enable it to function. Not surprisingly, some foods are better than others at forming these building blocks of life—particularly when it comes to brain health. So, it's important to eat healthy foods. That's easy to say, but which foods are healthy and which are not? Are grains like quinoa and whole wheat good for you or do they cause dementia? Is it true that eating red meat is unhealthy? Are berries as beneficial as people say? And what about vitamins and supplements? We'll discuss these issues and more in this chapter.

GENERAL PRINCIPLES

The first general principle is that your brain's health is directly related to the health of the rest of your body. So, it's critically important to eat foods that are good for the health of your heart, blood vessels, and other organs.

Second, it is important to maintain a healthy weight in the normal range for your height, which means a body mass index of 18.5 to 24.9. Not sure how to calculate your body mass index? There's a National Institutes of Health website that will do it for you.[1]

Third, whole, unprocessed foods with fewer ingredients are best.

Fourth, vitamins, antioxidants, and other nutrients are better from foods than pills, with the exception of vitamin D and the B vitamins.

Fifth, there is no single "superfood"—eating a balanced, Mediterranean-style menu of foods in moderation is best.

MEDITERRANEAN EATING

Over 7,500 articles have been published showing the benefits of eating a Mediterranean-style diet for reducing one's risk of cancer, diabetes, high blood pressure, high cholesterol, and heart disease in addition to brain health. Studies have shown that middle-aged adults who follow a Mediterranean style of eating are able to reduce their risk of Alzheimer's disease.[2] The MIND (Mediterranean-DASH [Dietary Approaches to Stop Hypertension] Intervention for Neurodegenerative Delay) diet has been shown to slow cognitive decline and reduce the incidence of Alzheimer's disease.[3,4] Other studies have shown that Mediterranean-style eating is beneficial for cognition in general, and that eating fish, in particular, is key.[5] One study showed that the brains of those who followed a Mediterranean diet appeared 5 years younger on magnetic resonance imaging

(MRI) scans.[4] The basic Mediterranean-style menu of foods includes:

- Fish
- Olive oil
- Avocados
- Vegetables
- Fruits
- Nuts
- Beans
- Whole grains (including bulgur, barley, and brown rice)

Based on the Mediterranean menu, the MIND diet includes:

- Olive oil daily
- Green leafy vegetables daily
- Other vegetables daily
- Whole grains daily
- Nuts and beans every other day
- Berries twice a week
- Poultry twice a week
- Fish once a week

Now you might be wondering: What about red wine, since that is traditionally part of Mediterranean-style eating? Stay tuned; we'll discuss wine and other alcoholic beverages in Chapter 19.

WHICH FISH IS BEST?

We've just recommended eating fish regularly. You may be wondering which fish is best to eat—and which to avoid because of possible high levels of mercury. Some of the good fish to eat with low levels of mercury include Atlantic mackerel, black sea bass, catfish, clams, cod, crab, crawfish, flounder, haddock, lobster, salmon, sardines, scallops, shrimp, skate, sole, squid,

tilapia, trout, and canned light tuna. Fish that may have particularly high levels of mercury include swordfish and bigeye
tuna; you would only want to eat these fish occasionally. The
U.S. Food and Drug Administration (FDA) has a good guide to
help you know which fish are best to eat.[6]

WHOLE GRAINS IN MODERATION ARE NOT HARMFUL

Whole grains are part of Mediterranean-style eating. Yet some
people think that eating any grains—even whole grains—are
bad for your brain. This idea comes from two truths.

First, consumption of refined grains is bad for you. When
grains are refined, the bran and germ are removed and the
grain loses nutritional value and fiber. The white flour or white
rice that remains is almost pure carbohydrate—complex sugars that are very quickly turned into simple sugars by your gut.
When these simple sugars are absorbed, they cause a spike in
blood sugar and insulin that is not good for the brain. Thus,
white bread, white rice, most pastas, and many cold cereals,
cakes, cookies, and pastries are not good for your brain health.

Second, people with celiac disease are allergic to gluten,
which is part of wheat. A number of studies have found that
those with celiac disease can show problems with memory and
thinking if, despite or not knowing about their allergy, they
consume gluten. Some individuals without celiac disease have
also noticed that they don't remember as well or think as clearly
when they consume gluten. We certainly agree that those with
celiac disease or known gluten sensitivity should not consume
wheat that contains gluten.

On the other hand, whole grains and foods made from them,
such as wheat and rye bread, oats, barley, brown rice, and quinoa, are rich in nutrients, are converted to sugar slowly, and
do not cause detrimental spikes in blood sugar. There is no

evidence that moderate consumptions of whole grains as part of a balanced, Mediterranean-style diet either impairs memory or leads to an increased risk of Alzheimer's disease or other cause of dementia.

OMEGA-3 FATTY ACIDS

One reason fish, walnuts, and green leafy vegetables are good for brain health is that they contain omega-3 fatty acids (often shortened to "omega-3s"). Although your body can make many of the fats you need, it cannot make omega-3s, and so you need to get them from food. There are three main types of omega-3s, which we will mention briefly (despite their long names).

1. Docosahexaenoic acid (DHA) has been associated with brain health and cognitive function, control of inflammation, as well as heart health.
2. Eicosapentaenoic acid (EPA) has been associated with heart health and control of inflammation.
3. Alpha-linoleic acid (ALA) is a source of energy and also a building block for both DHA and EPA.

Should you take omega-3 supplements? One study found that adults aged 18 to 45 taking about a gram of DHA daily for 6 months showed improvements in episodic and working memory,[7] but an accompanying editorial found serious problems with the study.[8] Although studies have suggested that low levels of DHA can increase one's risk of mild cognitive impairment or Alzheimer's disease,[9] a well-conducted study found that individuals with mild to moderate Alzheimer's disease showed no benefit from taking 2 grams of DHA daily.[10]

Based on these studies, our recommendation is not to take supplements, but to make sure your balanced diet does include some foods that contain omega-3 fatty acids. As mentioned, the most common sources of omega-3s include fish (particularly fatty fishes such as salmon and tuna), walnuts, green leafy vegetables (such as kale), as well as flaxseeds and flaxseed oil.

VITAMIN D

Vitamin D is essential for your brain health. If children don't receive enough vitamin D it can cause rickets, a disease that commonly affects bones and brain. Adults with low levels of vitamin D are about twice as likely to develop Alzheimer's disease compared with those whose levels are normal.[11] Many people don't have enough vitamin D. Although you can actually make this vitamin through your skin, you need to spend sufficient time outside without sunblock—which we don't recommend.

Because of how serious its deficiency is, vitamin D is one of the few nutrients that we recommend you take as a supplement pill. A daily dose of 2,000 IU of vitamin D_3 is the right amount for most people. You can also get vitamin D from fatty fish (such as salmon), portobello mushrooms grown under an ultraviolet light, and foods fortified with vitamin D, including milk, cereals, and orange juice. Note that there are some important interactions between vitamin D and certain prescription medications, so you should speak with your doctor prior to taking vitamin D supplements.

B VITAMINS

The B vitamins are another group in which supplements are sometimes helpful. As we mentioned in Chapter 14, low levels of vitamin B_{12} (cyanocobalamin) can cause depression, anxiety, and psychosis in addition to impairment of memory and thinking. Liver and clams have the most B_{12}, although fish and other shellfish, meats, milk, and yogurt also have some. Many people have trouble absorbing enough B_{12} from foods as they get older, but by taking a supplement as well (such as 250 or 500 micrograms daily) they can usually overcome this problem and get enough into their body. Some individuals, however, cannot absorb the vitamin at all and will need injections. The best way to determine if you need supplemental B_{12} pills or injections is to work with your doctor and get your level checked.

Thiamine (vitamin B_1) deficiency can cause a form of potentially reversible memory loss and confusion called Wernicke's encephalopathy, as well as a devastating, permanent loss of memory called Korsakoff syndrome (or Korsakoff amnesia), which is often associated with alcoholism. Thiamine-rich foods include whole grains, legumes, fruit, and yeast. However, if one has alcoholism, we recommend taking 100 milligrams of thiamine daily.

Although deficiencies of B_6 and folate (vitamin B_9) are uncommon, they can cause confusion and impaired memory, and are sometimes seen in the elderly and those with kidney problems, autoimmune disorders, and alcoholism. Low levels of B_6 and folate have also been associated with an increased risk of developing Alzheimer's disease. Foods rich in B_6 include chickpeas, tuna, salmon, potatoes, bananas, turkey, marinara sauce, beef, pistachios, and dark chocolate. Foods rich in folate include dark green leafy vegetables, fruits, nuts, beans, peas, seafood, eggs, dairy products, meat, poultry, and grains. You can also get B_6 and folate from a B-complex vitamin or separate pills. Note, however, that too much B_6 is highly toxic (it can cause a severe neuropathy), so we do not recommend more than 50 milligrams daily. For folate we do not recommend more than 1,000 micrograms daily, unless you are pregnant or planning to get pregnant (in which case you should speak with your doctor).

ONCE-IN-A-WHILE FOODS

Now that you know the foods that are good for you are on a Mediterranean-style menu, you may be wondering which foods are not so good for you. Which ones are they? Well . . . they're almost everything else. The following foods should be infrequently eaten:

- Red meats
- Butter and margarine
- Fried foods
- Fast foods
- Highly processed foods
- Pastries and sweets
- White bread, white flour, and white rice
- Most pasta
- Regular sodas and juices as well as diet sodas and juices with artificial sweeteners

Wondering what's wrong with diet sodas and juices? It turns out that the artificial sweeteners mimic sugar so well that they actually cause a spike in insulin in your body. This is detrimental for two reasons. The first is that these high insulin spikes are not good for the brain. The second is that the insulin spike makes you hungry, and you end up eating more than if you drank water without the artificial sweetener.

WHAT TO DRINK?

Speaking of water, plain water is one of the best beverages to drink with your food. If you prefer bubbles, soda/seltzer water is fine too. Coffee and tea—in moderation because of the caffeine—are also good to drink. Decaffeinated coffee and tea and herbal teas are a nice way to enjoy these drinks without the caffeine. Chilled water that is flavored with mint, other herbs, herbal teas, a bit of fruit, or even vegetables can be delicious and good for you. (We will discuss alcoholic beverages in Chapter 19.)

WHAT ABOUT DESSERT?

Some of you are probably thinking that, given the evidence, you should never eat dessert again. Not true! First, berries and other fruits are nutritious and make a terrific dessert. Second, chocolate, in small amounts, has been shown to benefit thinking, memory, and mood. Just remember that the benefit comes from the actual raw cocoa, so the darker the chocolate the better.

In the United States, dark chocolate has a minimum of 35% cocoa, sweet chocolate a minimum of 15%, and milk chocolate a minimum of 10%—meaning that even dark chocolate may not have a lot of cocoa in it. Look for the amount on the package; some dark chocolate is 60% to 90% cocoa. The recommended daily amount of chocolate is between 0.35 and 1.6 ounces, which is about one-third of a typical chocolate bar. Remember not to overdo it—chocolate is high in calories, fat, and sugar, and so too much of it can be detrimental to your health.

NUTRIENTS WITHOUT EVIDENCE

We wanted to mention a few of the diets, foods, and spices that are advocated for by some but that we don't recommend. Because fish and other seafood are so good for you, you might think that *fish oil* would be good for you too. Unfortunately, there are no studies to support supplementation with fish oil. Similarly, although some have claimed that *coconut oil* improves memory, brain health, and one's risk of Alzheimer's, there are no scientific studies to support such claims. *Ginkgo biloba* was also thought to be helpful, but subsequent studies showed no benefit on cognition or on reducing one's risk of cognitive decline, Alzheimer's disease, or other dementias.[12,13]

Resveratrol
Resveratrol is found in blueberries and red wine and was hypothesized to be the brain protective factor in those foods.

Because of this, a carefully conducted year-long study gave people with mild to moderate Alzheimer's disease 2,000 milligrams daily—the amount of resveratrol in 60 tons of blueberries or 186 bottles of red wine. Although resveratrol was safe and well tolerated, no clear beneficial effects were observed.[14] So, although it won't hurt you, we do not recommend resveratrol.

Curcumin

We love spicy curries and are always hoping to open our clinical and scientific journals to read about a large, well-conducted study showing that curcumin—one of the components in the curry spice turmeric—benefits memory, thinking, or brain health in any way. Unfortunately, such studies are still lacking. So, if you like spicy curry dishes—enjoy them. But we don't recommend adding more curries to your weekly menu to improve your memory given the available evidence at this time.

Ketogenic Diet

The ketogenic diet is a high-fat, low-carbohydrate, adequate-protein diet that has been successfully used to control seizures in some children whose epilepsy could not otherwise be controlled. Two small studies with 20 or fewer subjects have suggested that the ketogenic diet can improve memory or blood flow to the brain in individuals with Alzheimer's disease. Larger studies are needed, however, before we would recommend this diet. Although it can promote weight loss, which may be beneficial in some people, it also has serious side effects, including constipation, hypoglycemia (low blood sugar), elevated cholesterol, and kidney stones.

Prevagen

Prevagen is an over-the-counter supplement containing a protein found in jellyfish called apoaequorin. Its advertising boasts that it is "the leading memory support and brain health supplement in America," which certainly may be true given how much is sold. But does it work? Not at all. In fact, the U.S. Federal Trade Commission charged its makers with false and deceptive advertising.[15] Don't waste your money.

NEVER TOO LATE TO START EATING HEALTHY

Perhaps by now we've convinced you that eating a Mediterranean-style menu of whole, minimally processed foods is good for you and your memory. Are you worried that you're too old for a change in your eating to improve your brain health? The good news is that it's not too late. One study found that even 55- to 80-year-old adults showed benefits by switching to a Mediterranean menu.[16]

YOU DON'T HAVE TO BE PERFECT

Don't worry about trying to be perfect. There is ample evidence that just making some healthy choices regarding what you eat will benefit your memory and thinking and reduce your risk of Alzheimer's disease. For example, although those who followed the MIND diet (described earlier in this chapter) "rigorously" showed a 53% reduction in their risk of developing Alzheimer's disease, those who followed the diet "moderately well" still showed a 35% reduction in risk—quite a large amount.[4]

EAT HEALTHY ON A BUDGET

Want to eat healthy on a budget? Here are a few tips.

- Buy the fresh fruits and vegetables that are in season; they'll be less expensive and more likely to be locally produced.
- Buy local fish (if available); it will likely be less expensive and fresher.

- Buy store brands.
- To avoid expensive and unhealthy impulse buys, shop using a list and don't go to the grocery store hungry.
- Buy enough ingredients to cook more than one meal and refrigerate or freeze additional portions for another night.

EAT FOR BRAIN HEALTH

Keep your memory strong by providing your body with good nutrition.

- Maintain a healthy weight in the normal range for your height, which means a body mass index of 18.5 to 24.9.
- Eat a Mediterranean menu of foods: fish, olive oil, avocados, vegetables, fruits, berries, nuts, beans, whole grains, and poultry.
- Foods to be eaten rarely include red meats, butter, margarine, fried foods, fast foods, highly processed foods, pastries, sweets, white bread, white flour, white rice, most pasta, regular sodas, diet sodas, and juices.

19

This is your brain on alcohol, cannabis, and drugs

You open your eyes slowly and look around in the dim light, seeing empty bottles of beer, wine, and liquor littering the floor. Your gaze falls on the nightstand covered with drug paraphernalia, empty bags, and crumpled papers. As you continue to look around, you realize that you have no idea where you are, how you got there, or anything that happened last night. You can remember getting ready for the party, but everything is a haze after that. You wonder what you might have drunk, smoked, snorted, ingested, or injected that left you with such a hole in your memory.

We hope you've never had an experience like this one, a "blackout" period when you couldn't remember anything. As we will discuss, alcohol, cannabis, and drugs (both legal and illegal) can impair your memory. Their effects are typically more subtle than the complete blackout in our story, but they are every bit as real. In this chapter we'll review the data to answer questions such as: Should you drink red wine or abstain from alcohol? Does cannabis help your memory or harm it? Are illegal drugs as bad as those old television messages—"This is your brain on drugs?"—or is that all hype?

ALCOHOL

Have you experienced difficulty remembering information, perhaps someone's name, after a drink or two? Although there are individual differences between one person and another, it is well established that alcohol interferes with both procedural memory and episodic memory.

Procedural Memory

While you might first think of party games such as "beer pong" when considering how alcohol interferes with procedural memory (Chapter 2), probably the most important—and terrible—example is the fact that drunk drivers are involved in one-quarter of all motor vehicle fatalities. Procedural memory is critical for your reaction time, your routine driving actions such as turns and lane changes, and your automatic responses to situations such as the car in front of you suddenly slowing down. Alcohol disrupts several brain regions critical for procedural memory, including the cerebellum (the "little brain" in the back and bottom part of your head). In fact, when used habitually, alcohol can damage the cerebellum—permanently impairing procedural memory.

Episodic Memory

Alcohol's effects on episodic memory are especially notable during the encoding (learning) process. Individuals who drink too much alcohol in an evening can experience alcoholic blackouts in which they wake up the next morning not remembering what happened the night before. But less alcohol consumption can also interfere with learning and memory.

In order to understand more about how alcohol interferes with learning, a group of researchers in Toronto put healthy young adults into a magnetic resonance imaging (MRI) scanner after consuming orange juice spiked with either a large amount of alcohol (the "alcohol group") or just enough alcohol to taste it (the "placebo group"). While their brains were being scanned, both groups had to learn pairs of objects and names of people. The researchers found that, after consuming alcohol, parts of the prefrontal cortex (your *central executive*, see Chapters 3 and 4) were less active, as were regions neighboring the hippocampus—all brain areas typically active when you are building your memories (see Part 2). Perhaps not surprisingly, when they were tested 24 hours later outside of the scanner, memory for both the pairs of objects and the names of people was impaired in the alcohol group compared to the placebo group.[1]

In another study, college students learned some information on day 1 to about 90% accuracy. The participants were then divided into three groups. The control group had their memory tested on day 7; they were still about 90% accurate. The members of the second group were given enough alcohol to make them a little drunk just before bed on day 1; on day 7 their memory accuracy dropped below 50%. The members of the third group were given enough alcohol to make them a little drunk just before bed on day 3; by day 7 their memory accuracy dropped to about 60%. This surprising result means that not only will alcohol interfere with your memory when you are intoxicated, but it will also interfere with your retention of information you learned earlier in the day—or earlier in the week. Why is this the case? Because alcohol interferes with sleep, and sleep—as we will discuss in Chapter 20—plays a critical role in memory.

Is Drinking in Moderation Good or Bad?

So, alcohol interferes with memory function—you knew that already, right? But is drinking in moderation good for the brain? After all, red wine is a traditional part of the Mediterranean menu. Some studies have, in fact, found that one alcoholic beverage daily can reduce one's risk of dementia.[2] Other papers, however, have questioned this finding, suggesting that some of the prior studies showing a benefit of alcohol consumption on dementia risk were flawed.[3] An extensive review of the available data on alcohol consumption found that it is the leading risk factor for disease burden worldwide, noting that "the safest level of drinking is none."[4] Some researchers have suggested that the small correlations observed between moderate drinking and health are attributable to the fact that when people become ill they generally stop drinking, arguing that it isn't that drinking keeps you healthy, it's just that unhealthy people don't drink.

Our Recommendations

First, don't fool yourself. Whether it is a 12-ounce beer, a 5-ounce glass of wine, or 1 ounce of liquor in a cocktail, even a single alcoholic drink will impair your episodic and procedural memory to some degree. That doesn't mean you shouldn't have one, but if you are trying to learn the names of a dozen people you're meeting in a party, you'll be more likely to remember them if you don't drink. You'll also be more likely to remember information you learned during the week if you don't get drunk on the weekend. And do not have more than one drink and drive or engage in other procedural memory tasks where safety is an issue, such as biking or downhill skiing. (No one should have more than one drink in these circumstances, but note that everyone's tolerance for alcohol is different. Know yourself. Some people will be impaired drivers after a single drink.)

Second, our reading of the clinical and scientific literature is that a single alcoholic beverage daily neither helps nor harms your brain. So, if you enjoy a glass of wine with dinner or a beer with the ballgame, go right ahead. However, we would strongly recommend limiting yourself to no more than two drinks per day and seven in a given week.

Third, we would never recommend that you start drinking for your health. If you currently abstain, there is no evidence that starting to drink will benefit your brain.

Lastly, if you have a history of drinking problems, don't drink.

CANNABIS

Cannabis (also known as marijuana) is now legal for recreational use in more than a dozen U.S. states and is legal in some form for medical use in all but two. It is also legal for recreational use in Canada and several other countries, and decriminalized or otherwise tolerated in almost 50 others. Does this mean science has shown that it does not impair brain function? Unfortunately not. As we learned with alcohol (and junk food), the legality of a substance does not mean that it is good for you.

Procedural Memory

Does using cannabis impair procedural memory? As we discussed earlier, the most important procedural memory task you do is driving. Although several early studies suggested that cannabis users can functionally compensate for their intoxication and drive more cautiously,[5] more recent studies have found that the proportion of cannabis-positive drivers involved in fatal crashes has dramatically increased with legalization. For example, in Washington state the percentage of drivers involved in fatal crashes who tested positive for cannabis rose from 9% to 18%.[6] This statistic should be viewed with caution, however, because non-intoxicated cannabis users may test positive for several weeks. Nonetheless, acute cannabis intoxication is associated with an increased number of collisions, increased lateral movement such as lane weaving, increased brake latency, and slower reaction time.[7] To summarize, cannabis impairs procedural memory.

Episodic Memory

Some of the prior research on cannabis and its users had been potentially confounded by the fact that there are usually a number of differences between individuals who chronically use cannabis and nonusers, in addition to their use of cannabis. It therefore makes it difficult to compare those populations directly. Researchers at Massachusetts General Hospital in Boston, however, conducted a clever experiment to get around this problem. They invited 88 cannabis users aged 16 to 25 into a study, tested their attention and episodic memory, and then randomly assigned two-thirds of them to stop using cannabis for a month, while the other one-third continued to use it. Use and cessation were monitored by urine tests. The results were clear: Cannabis cessation did not have an effect on attention, but it did have a significant beneficial effect on episodic memory—particularly during the encoding (learning) of material.[8] Given that 16- to 25-year-olds are often in school and need to be learning new material, this is an important finding. A similar increase in episodic memory was observed in 30- to 55-year-old users when they ceased cannabis use for 28 days.[9] Additionally, a meta-analysis that combined six studies found that compared to nonusers, cannabis users were impaired in prospective memory—the ability to remember to carry out intended actions in the future.[10] So, it is clear that cannabis impairs episodic memory, but memory function appears to return to normal with cessation of cannabis use.

THC Versus CBD

Two of the many compounds in cannabis are $\Delta 9$-tetrahydrocannabinol and cannabidiol, known better as THC and CBD, respectively. It is primarily intoxication with THC that produces the subjective feeling of being "stoned" and impairs memory.[11] Several studies (although not all) have found that CBD may be able to improve episodic memory in individuals with acute THC intoxication.[11,12] So, in theory, the CBD in cannabis might be able to reverse its THC-induced memory-impairing effects. Unfortunately, while that might have been true in the 1990s, when the ratio of the average concentrations of THC to CBD in cannabis were about 15 to 1, the ratio in today's cannabis may exceed 80 to 1.[13] This means there's not enough CBD in most current strains of cannabis to counteract its memory-impairing effects.

To shed light on this issue, researcher Carrie Cuttler and her colleagues at Washington State University asked participants to use one of several cannabis strains with different percentages of THC, with or without CBD. They found that all strains of cannabis impaired some aspect of memory commonly used in everyday life, such as remembering a list off the top of your head or recalling where you learned a bit of information. Interestingly, the ability to distinguish true from false memories also was impaired by all strains.[14]

Can CBD improve memory in individuals who are not intoxicated by THC? Researchers at the University of Basel, Switzerland, set out to answer this question by asking 34 healthy young adults to participate in two conditions. In each condition they learned a list of 15 unrelated nouns; this was followed by vaping either 12.5 mg of CBD or a similarly flavored placebo. Participants remembered slightly more words in the CBD condition (7.7 words) compared to the placebo condition (7.0 words).[15] Not a terribly huge effect or large study, but certainly intriguing and worthy of further research.

Given that CBD may be able to improve memory in healthy young adults, some people have wondered if CBD can help memory impairment in conditions such as Alzheimer's disease. Although researchers are looking into this possibility, to date no studies have found that CBD produces improvement in memory or any other cognitive function in individuals with Alzheimer's. And, for what it's worth, when Andrew's patients with Alzheimer's disease or their families have asked him whether they should try CBD, he always encourages them to do so and let him know if it helps. Thus far, none have reported any beneficial effects in memory, mood, or anxiety. But none have reported any adverse effects of CBD on memory either, consistent with the published studies.

Some Thoughts on Cannabis Use

It is our job to interpret the data that make up the science of memory as we see it and present these findings to you. It is up to you, of course, to determine how such findings fit into your life. Cannabis has many documented medical uses. In fact, it was added to the U.S. Pharmacopeia in 1850 and remained there until 1942—when it was removed for political rather than scientific reasons. We view cannabis like any other medication, with beneficial effects and side effects. We believe the data is clear that the THC in cannabis interferes with procedural and episodic memory, just like alcohol and the more than 100 approved drugs we discussed in Chapter 14 and listed in the Appendix. Just like these other medications, cannabis may be the best option for your chronic pain or other medical problem, despite its effects on your memory. (In fact, one study showed that some aspects of thinking improved after initiation of medical cannabis, which the researchers speculated may have been attributable to participants' decreased use of prescription medications known to impair memory and thinking—opioids, benzodiazepines, anticholinergic antidepressants, and mood stabilizers like valproic acid; see the Appendix.[16]) Whether used recreationally or for medical purposes, you now know that cannabis will likely impair your driving, your memory for new information, and your ability to remember to act in the future. So, if you do use cannabis, as with alcohol, we would simply recommend that you do so responsibly.

DRUGS

Cocaine

Although much could be said about cocaine's effect on memory, here we would like to highlight that cocaine predisposes you to strokes. It raises your blood pressure, causes your blood vessels to constrict, and disrupts normal heart function. There are many individuals with memory impairment—and full-blown vascular dementia—due to cocaine-induced strokes. Many of these individuals were in their 20s and 30s when they had their strokes. See Chapters 13 and 14 to learn more about strokes and vascular dementia.

Ecstasy

Ecstasy (MDMA or 3,4-methylenedioxymethamphetamine, also known as Molly) is a recreational drug that has been gaining in popularity. Ecstasy users show both working and episodic memory impairments compared with nonusers. Interestingly, their episodic memory for verbal information was particularly impaired, as was their prospective memory.[10,17] These impairments in episodic memory may be related to the diminished hippocampal activation observed in Ecstasy users.[18]

Methamphetamine

When used properly as a medication, stimulant drugs such as methylphenidate (brand name Ritalin as well as others) and amphetamine/dextroamphetamine (brand name Adderall as well as others) can improve both working and episodic memory in individuals with attention-deficit/hyperactivity disorder (ADHD). Methamphetamine (brand names Desoxyn and Methedrine) can also be used to treat ADHD as well as obesity, but it is more commonly used as a recreational drug. Despite its ability to boost memory when used properly, recreational methamphetamine users show impairments in their episodic memory, including their prospective memory, compared with nonusers.[10,19]

Opioids

When fentanyl, heroin, Percocet, oxycodone, or other opioids are used—whether for prescribed pain management, for recreational purposes, or because of addiction—they also cause memory impairment and confusion. The good news is that not only will memory improve with abstinence, it will also improve with maintenance treatment with the less harmful opioid, methadone.[20] So, if you or a loved one are suffering from memory problems due to opioid use, we recommend you seek treatment today. You'll improve your memory—and your life.

Psychedelics

Classic psychedelic drugs include lysergic acid diethylamide (LSD), mescaline (the active chemical in peyote), psilocybin (the active ingredient in psychedelic mushrooms), and *N,N*-dimethyltryptamine (DMT, the primary hallucinogenic chemical in the Amazonian brew *ayahuasca* or *yagé*). These drugs have been used in the past by clinicians to facilitate individuals' ability to recall childhood experiences from memory. It is therefore reasonable to consider whether such drugs may be beneficial to memory.

The scientific studies, however, clearly show dose-dependent impairment in working memory, semantic memory, and non-autobiographical episodic memory, such that low doses cause some impairment and higher doses cause greater impairment.[21] The retrieval of autobiographical episodic memory may be facilitated, but it is generally only observed in individuals who have suppressed and/or unpleasant memories, such that the mechanism of this facilitation is thought to be disruption of inhibitory control processes. Lastly, it should be noted that individuals may be more likely to experience false memories under the influence of psychedelics, as memories of aliens, angels, and elves are not uncommon. So, even when retrieval of autobiographical episodic memories is facilitated with psychedelics, the accuracy of these memories may be unreliable.

YOUR BRAIN ON ALCOHOL, CANNABIS, AND DRUGS

Know the effects of substances on your memory:

- Even a single alcoholic beverage will interfere with procedural memory (for example, driving) and episodic memory (for example, remembering new facts and events of your life).
  - Drinking alcohol will interfere with your retention of information you learned earlier in the day—and earlier in the week.
  - As an adult, consuming one alcoholic beverage each day should not permanently damage your brain, but there also is no reason to drink in an effort to improve your brain health.
- Using cannabis will impair your procedural and episodic memory.
  - CBD alone does not impair memory—and may even help it.
  - Cannabis has not been shown to permanently damage memory.
- Cocaine, Ecstasy, methamphetamine, opioids, and psychedelics will all impair your memory.
  - Cocaine can cause strokes—even in young people—and may lead to vascular dementia and life-long consequences for memory.

20

Sleep well

You've always been good at languages, and so, entering college, you decide you're going to take two new ones, German and Arabic. You're a planner, and you've mapped out your studying for the whole semester. You allocate equal studying time for each. For Arabic, in addition to class, you plan to study for 1 hour on Mondays, Tuesdays, Wednesdays, and Thursdays during the 10-week semester, totaling 40 hours. The German midterm and final, however, are each scheduled right when you return from vacation. You know the material will be fresher in your mind if you study right before the exams, so, in addition to class, you plan to study 10 hours a day on the 2 days prior to the midterm, and the same for the final, also totaling 40 hours. The semester starts and you follow your plan. To your delight, you receive straight A's in both midterms and both finals. Returning to college in your sophomore year, sitting in the second-year classes for each language, you discover that you retained one of these languages quite well, while the other has almost completely vanished.

Which language was retained, and which vanished? And why did it happen like that? We will answer these and related questions in this chapter. The preview, as you no doubt have guessed, is that it is related to your sleep. Sleep is absolutely critical for normal memory function.

IT'S HARD TO PAY ATTENTION WHEN YOU'RE TIRED

The first reason that sleep is important for memory is the obvious one. As you learned in Parts 1 and 2, in order to learn new information so it can be remembered, you need to pay attention to the information! And we all know that it is hard to pay attention when you're tired. This is one of many reasons why it is not beneficial to stay up all night studying—because your tired brain will do a poor job of encoding the information you're trying to learn.

Two Drives to Sleep

Why do we get tired? Sleep is determined by two drives.

Sleep pressure (also called sleep debt) builds up while you are awake; the longer you are awake, the greater the pressure you feel to sleep. Sleep pressure is related to the accumulation of certain chemicals in your brain, whose levels return to normal when you sleep.

Circadian rhythm governs your normal, daily patterns of sleep and wakefulness; it is why you may wake up before your alarm goes off and why you suffer from jet lag. Your circadian rhythm is primarily set by the light you see during the day, which triggers the release of *melatonin* hours later. Melatonin is a hormone that tells your brain it is time to begin the process to go to sleep.

You become tired either when your sleep pressure builds up to sufficient levels or when your circadian rhythm has triggered the release of melatonin indicating it is time to sleep. When your sleep routine is consistent, these two drives are in sync, such that when it is time for you to go to sleep, your sleep pressure is at its maximum and your melatonin levels are rising rapidly. If, however, these drives are divergent, you will still feel tired from either one—and you'll have difficulty learning new information.

For example, let's say that you're flying from Boston to London. You take a flight that leaves at 8:30 p.m. and, due to your hectic day preparing for your trip, you fall asleep before the flight even takes off. You wake up when the plane lands 6.5 hours later. Although it's 8 a.m. London time and 6.5 hours is long enough to relieve your sleep pressure, you find you're dead tired. Why? Because according to your circadian rhythm it's 3 in the morning Boston time and you should be fast asleep.

Another time you're at home and not changing time zones, but you've just finished pulling an all-nighter for work. It's 8 a.m. and your circadian rhythm is ready for you to be awake for another day, but you're exhausted because your sleep pressure has been building up for more than 24 hours.

Does Caffeine Help?

So, let's say you're tired because of either mounting sleep pressure from staying up too late, or because your circadian rhythm is out of whack from sleeping till noon every day of your week-long vacation and now you're back at work 8 a.m. Monday morning. Will it help if you drink a cup of coffee, tea, or an energy drink with a shot of caffeine in it?

The answer, as you may know from your own experience, is yes and no. Caffeine temporarily blocks the effects of sleep pressure and can restore a level of alertness needed to adequately pay attention so you can remember information. However, caffeine can only do so much in the face of mounting sleep pressure. The bottom line is that caffeine can help you be more alert for a time, but it is no substitute for keeping a constant circadian rhythm and getting a good night's sleep. Which leads us to the next reason as to why sleep is important for memory.

SLEEP TO GET READY FOR NEW LEARNING

Remember the hippocampus, the part of your brain shaped like a seahorse that is involved in the storage, retention, and retrieval of memories discussed in Parts 1 and 2? It has a limited number of cells that must be used to store new memories. Exceed that limit and you may not be able to keep new information distinct from already-learned information—or you may overwrite one memory with another. Have you ever been studying the same type of material for hours on end and find that details of some facts start to get confused with that of other facts until much of what you're trying to learn seems to be melting together? That may be a sign that you've reached your capacity for remembering that type of information—until you sleep.

As you learned in Chapter 4, when you sleep you are able to shift major responsibilities for retrieval of your recently acquired memories from your hippocampus to your cortex (the outer layers of the brain) where those memories can have more permanent, long-term storage. If the memory is about you, it will likely still contain a link to the hippocampus. If, however, the memory is for facts—such as who Rosa Parks was—the connection to the hippocampus can be severed without diminishing the accuracy of this semantic memory (see Chapter 5). In either case, you have succeeded in freeing up hippocampal capacity, so you wake with refreshed ability for new learning (Figure 20.1, top).

THE SHRINKING BRAIN

How do you free up brain capacity? There's evidence that about 80% of the brain's synapses—the connections between neurons—shrink while we sleep. Smaller connections indicate that the strength of memory traces is reduced or eliminated entirely. This shrinkage is selective, such that the most stable (presumably important) memory traces remain unaffected while most other connections shrink to get ready for new learning. This is thought to be one of the mechanisms of how, over

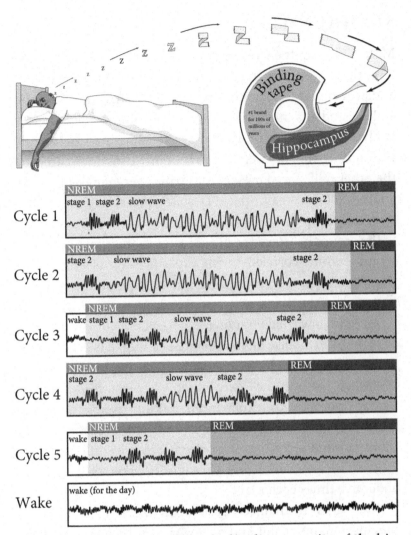

Figure 20.1. Sleep replenishes the binding capacity of the hippocampus (top). EEG waveforms of typical sleep cycles across a night's sleep (bottom).

time, we forget unimportant things that happened to us during the previous day yet still remember the important things.[1] This model of memory selectivity is, however, not the only one. Reactivation of important memories during sleep is also critical, as we will discuss.

STAGES OF SLEEP

Matt Walker, at the University of California at Berkeley, helped to both demonstrate the importance of sleep for new learning and provide evidence for one part of its mechanism. He invited college students into his laboratory and, at noon, had them all study 100 faces, each of which was paired with a unique name. Half of the students were then randomly chosen to nap, while the other half stayed awake. At 6 p.m., everyone tried to learn another 100 face–name pairs. Despite equal ability to pay attention, the group that napped learned 20% more pairs compared to the group that stayed awake. Moreover, this increased capacity for learning correlated with a specific stage of sleep. Which stage is most important? To answer this question, we need to first explain the different stages of sleep.[2]

As you know from your own experience, if you are woken up at night from a noise or your bladder calling, it is usually when you are sleeping lightly or perhaps dreaming, and only rarely is it when you are in a "deep" sleep when you feel dead tired. Perhaps you've only experienced waking from a deep sleep when you are jet-lagged. In any event, you probably have an intuitive experience that your sleep occurs in different stages. In fact, we generally cycle through different stages of sleep about five times each night.

The stages are named based upon whether your eyes are moving rapidly or not and also what can be seen on an electroencephalogram (EEG) if you have electrodes on your head recording your brain activity while you are sleeping. Rapid-eye-movement (REM) sleep is the stage when you have your most vigorous—and often bizarre—dreams. Non-REM (NREM) sleep is divided into stages 1, 2, 3, and 4. Stages 3 and 4 are usually grouped together and referred to as "slow-wave sleep," because during those stages your brain cells are firing in synchronous waves, creating "slow waves" on the EEG. Slow-wave sleep is "deep" sleep when you are hard to awaken, NREM stage

2 is "lighter" because you are easier to waken, and stage 1 is lighter still—so light that you may not even realize you were asleep if awakened from it.

Figure 20.1 (bottom) shows some typical sleep cycles across a normal night of sleep. You can see how the proportion of time spent in different cycles varies across the night. Note also that it is normal to briefly wake a couple of times each night, although you may not recall these awakenings.

Returning to Matt Walker's experiment with college students learning face–name pairs, he found that when the students were napping it was specifically the amount of time they spent in NREM stage 2 that was beneficial for learning more pairs. NREM stage 2 sleep contains bursts of activity called sleep "spindles" because of how they look on EEG. In fact, the number of sleep spindles themselves correlated with students' ability to learn more face–name pairs. This finding and others like it suggest that these spindles may help memories to be processed so as to avoid them from being forgotten.

CONSOLIDATE MEMORIES WHILE YOU SLEEP

You now understand another reason that sleep is so important to memory—it allows you to consolidate your memories, transferring them from transiently-accessible memories to those that can be recalled days or even years later. As we discussed in Chapters 4 and 5, many episodic memories that represent events of your life will still have a connection to the hippocampus, whereas most semantic memories for facts and information will be stored in the cortex alone.

This sleep-dependent consolidation process doesn't only free up the hippocampus for additional new learning but also helps to solidify the information you've learned in your memory. For example, if you learn a list of facts in the evening and then sleep for 8 hours, you could remember 20% to 40% more of them than if you learned that list in the morning and were awake for 8 hours. Moreover, the number of facts you will remember overnight correlates with your total time in NREM sleep.[3] Reviewing information you're hoping to commit to memory at night, soon before you sleep, can be a powerful tool to help you retain newly-learned information.

Your procedural memories—your memory for learned skills such as basketball and skiing—also become consolidated when you sleep. While you sleep, your brain is rehearsing the sequence of motor commands needed to perform an action. Sometimes, this means that you can wake up better at a motor skill than you were when you went to sleep. As we discussed in Chapter 2, although this "offline" learning can occur while you are awake, it is more robust when you are sleeping—and in particular, when you are in stage 2 NREM sleep. Because stage 2 NREM sleep is most prevalent at the end of sleep, athletes may not be helping themselves when they get up early to practice if to do so they are reducing their sleep by an hour or more. Basketball player LeBron James, for example, understands the importance of sleep to his performance: He sleeps 8 to 9 hours at night and may nap throughout the day for a few more hours.

SLEEP TO REMEMBER WHAT IS IMPORTANT

Sleep doesn't indiscriminately retain all memories—NREM sleep preferentially boosts the long-term memories that your brain has tagged as important in some way. Memories that are not important—such as what you had for breakfast this morning—will not be strengthened and, after a few nights of sleep, are likely to be forgotten altogether. Return to Parts 1 and 2 for why some memories are tagged as important and some are not.

CAN YOU USE SLEEP TO ENHANCE PARTICULAR MEMORIES?

If NREM sleep is so beneficial for memory, you may wonder if there are any ways to enhance some of the particular content you learned that day while you sleep.

Ken Paller and his colleagues at Northwestern University tested this idea by teaching participants to associate 50 unique object images with 50 specific locations on a computer screen. Each image was paired with its related sound, such as *meow* with cat. Participants then napped while listening to 25 of the paired sounds during NREM sleep. These sounds were played quite softly, to avoid awakening the participants. After the nap, participants were asked to use the computer mouse to move each object image to its specific location on the computer screen that they learned prior to their nap. Ten of 12 participants showed more accurate placement for the objects whose sound was presented while sleeping compared with the non-presented objects. Note that participants were unaware that they were presented with sounds while they were napping and were, in fact, at chance when asked to guess which sounds were presented while they slept.[4] There have now been over 90 experiments with more than 2,000 subjects confirming that replaying cues during both stage 2 NREM and slow-wave sleep works to improve memory for the cued material, including odors, sounds, and vocabulary words.[5]

So, should you start recording information you want to remember better and play it back while you are sleeping? Or should you try to enhance your memory more generally for information that was learned while listening to specific music or smelling specific odors by having that music or odor with you while you are sleeping? Perhaps. Experiments looking at the practical application of these types of techniques are currently ongoing and may lead to new ways to boost your memory.

INTERCONNECTING MEMORIES: REM SLEEP

You may have noticed that, thus far, we have mainly discussed the role of NREM sleep in memory. But REM sleep is important too. One intriguing hypothesis suggests that it is during REM sleep when your newly consolidated memories become interconnected with all of your prior memories, including your autobiographical life history and your storehouse of facts and knowledge.

If we ask you to think of the first word that comes to mind when we say "dream" you might think "sleep," and if we say "doctor" you might think "nurse," as sleep and nurse are strong associations for dream and doctor, respectively. But when Robert Stickgold and colleagues at Harvard University woke participants from REM sleep, they found that—judging by how quickly participants responded to different word pairs—weak associations were actually more accessible than strong associations. Participants awakened from REM were more likely to associate words with weak associations—such as "dream" with "sweet" and "doctor" with "office"—than they were to associate words with strong associations. It's as if, during REM sleep, the brain has an opportunity to try out different associations, and to see if any of them provide useful new insights. Often, they don't—although they may lead to strange dreams. But, as we talked about in Chapter 10, the ability to notice associations between different memories is critical for making new inferences, and so, sometimes, these weak connections highlighted in REM sleep provide an important new perspective on a problem.

Following up on these ideas, Kristin Sanders and colleagues at Northwestern University found that when participants were presented with puzzles in the evening, 20% of the unsolved puzzles could be solved the next morning. Although we consider this percentage by itself an impressive display of the power of sleep, participants were able to solve an additional 10% of unsolved puzzles if they were cued by being exposed to a sound related to the puzzle while they slept.[6] This experiment demonstrates not only the ability of sleep to help you solve problems, but also the importance of memory reactivation in finding the solution.

The most cited historical example of such creative problem-solving work while sleeping is that of Dmitri Mendeleev, who dreamed on February 17, 1869, where all the atomic elements should be placed in the periodic table—something he was unable to do for months while awake. Writing them down as soon as he awoke, he only needed to make one correction to the solution provided by his dream. Perhaps you, too, have been puzzling over a problem that your waking brain has been struggling to solve. As you are lying down with your eyes closed preparing yourself for sleep, spend a minute or two thinking about your problem. You just might wake up the next morning with the answer.

YOU'LL FEEL BETTER IN THE MORNING

Have you had the experience of being upset, and someone tells you, "Don't worry, you'll feel better in the morning"? When you woke the next day, did you feel better? We bet you did. In fact, we would guess that you continued to feel a little bit better each morning. Your experience of "feeling better" is related to a few functions of sleep. One is as we just described: Sleep can help you to gain a new perspective on a problem. You may fall asleep dreading a conversation you need to have with a coworker the next day. But in the morning, you may realize that you can use an experience from years ago—when you were on the receiving end of a critique from a boss—to help you constructively guide the conversation.

Another important function of sleep is to strip off the emotions related to painful, upsetting memories, while still keeping the memory content. In this way you still very clearly remember what upset you but, with sleep, you don't re-experience the full emotional intensity of the event every time you retrieve it from memory.

We again turn to a study by Matt Walker to help us understand how this stripping away of emotions occurs while you are sleeping. He had individuals view emotional photos while in an MRI scanner to monitor their brain activity. As expected, there was strong activation in the amygdala, an almond-shaped structure just in front of the hippocampus that generates emotions. All participants returned to the scanner 12 hours later, but half of the subjects were initially tested at night and therefore had a night's sleep between sessions, whereas the other half were initially tested in the morning and so were awake between the sessions. The researchers found that those who slept—but not those who were awake—had significant reductions in their emotional feelings as well as amygdala reactivation. Moreover, these important reductions correlated with the amount of time spent in REM sleep, suggesting that this is another important function of this stage of sleep.[3]

A related study by Rick Wassing and colleagues in Amsterdam found that not only is REM sleep important for this amygdala adaptation, but that the REM sleep needs to be relatively continuous with few interruptions for the adaptation to be successful. Participants whose REM sleep was highly fragmented did not show the beneficial emotion-reducing effects of sleep.[7]

Another researcher, Rosalind Cartwright at Rush University, found that it was critical for the dream itself to relate to the painful experience in order for individuals with depression to strip off the painful emotions and get past those experiences. Individuals who did not dream about their painful, traumatic experience could not remove the emotions from the event and did not experience remission of their depression.[8]

You may recall circumstances in which you dreamed—perhaps for several nights—about an upsetting event, only to feel somewhat better about it in the days and weeks that followed. Andrew has had this experience related to the most painful and traumatic experience of his life, that of his son Danny being diagnosed with severe autism before age 2. Danny never learned to talk. And so, the dreams that Andrew had, with variations for weeks and months, involved Danny talking. Andrew still feels sad on occasion when thinking of what might have been without the autism. But, likely because of these dreams, Andrew has been able to move past the pain of Danny's limitations and enjoy Danny's strengths and the time they spend together.

SLEEP TO REDUCE YOUR RISK OF ALZHEIMER'S DISEASE

In Chapter 13 we mentioned how Alzheimer's disease is caused by amyloid plaques and neurofibrillary tangles, collections of proteins that can be seen under the microscope. Most researchers believe that the disease starts with the amyloid plaques. Then, when the plaques get large enough, they begin to damage neighboring brain cells, which then form tangles—killing the cells.

It turns out that we all make some of this amyloid protein during the day. The normal function of amyloid is not clear; some researchers (including Andrew) believe it is involved in the brain's defense against infections. Although some amyloid may therefore be beneficial, too much is thought to directly cause Alzheimer's disease. How does our body get rid of excess amyloid so we don't all develop Alzheimer's? By sleeping, of course.

Maiken Nedergaard at the University of Rochester has done pioneering work on the brain's drainage mechanism, called the "glymphatic system." Although this system is active during the day, it is 10 to 20 times more active at night. So, we need our sleep to clear away excess amyloid protein.

As you might expect, there are studies that show you are at increased risk of dementia and Alzheimer's disease if you sleep poorly.[9,10] But there are also studies that show you can reduce your risk of Alzheimer's disease by improving your sleep.[11]

SLEEP TO REDUCE YOUR RISKS OF STROKES AND VASCULAR DEMENTIA

After Alzheimer's disease, strokes are the most common cause of memory loss and dementia. Insufficient sleep increases your risk of weight gain, high blood pressure, diabetes, and heart disease—all of which increase your risk of strokes, memory loss, and dementia, as discussed in more detail in Chapters 13 and 14.

DON'T PULL AN ALL-NIGHTER

It should be obvious by now that sleep is so important for memory and your brain that you're only going to decrease your performance on your test the next day if you "pull an all-nighter" and stay up all night. In addition to being tired the next day, leading to difficulty paying attention, when you are sleep deprived you'll retain less of the information you learned the previous day and will be much less able to learn new facts compared to having a good night's sleep.

Can you just catch up on your sleep on the weekend? No. Sleep isn't like a bank that you can borrow from and pay it back later. Of course, if life circumstances prevent you from getting enough sleep during the week (perhaps you are a new parent or working multiple shifts), then—by all means—take a nap when you can and try to go to sleep a bit earlier on the nights when it's possible for you to do so. There is some evidence that sleeping a little extra on the day prior to a late night can help your brain to function better. But, for ideal memory function, it is important to prioritize sleeping soundly each night.[12]

SLEEP AND SCHOOL

Now there are some individuals who routinely flout healthy sleep guidelines: They stay up late, get up early, and try to catch up on their sleep during the weekends. Who are these dangerous rulebreakers? Students, of course—particularly teenagers.

Although we've introduced this topic in a humorous way, student sleep is no laughing matter. Sleep has been studied in students in elementary school, middle school, high school, college, and medical school. In each and every case, the students who slept better performed better in school academically.[13,14]

Importantly, one study from researchers at the Massachusetts Institute of Technology measured sleep and test performance in college students during the month, week, and night prior to a test. Interestingly, although they found no relation between test performance and sleep the night before a test, they found a strong relation between sleep quality and test performance in the month and week before. This beneficial effect of sleep was so strong that it accounted for almost one-quarter of the differences observed between the grades in the class.[15] This and other studies like it make the point that good sleep habits over time really do make a difference in learning.

Speaking of school, students perform remarkably better when school start times are pushed back from 7:30 to 8:30 a.m. or later. Adolescence is a period of development associated with a circadian shift toward later sleep-onset times and later awakenings, and so shifting school start times can bring them into better alignment with teenagers' natural circadian rhythms. In one example from Edina, Minnesota, after shifting from a 7:25 a.m. to an 8:30 a.m. start time, verbal and mathematics Scholastic Aptitude Test (SAT) scores increased from 605 and

683 to 761 and 739, respectively.³ Petition your school district today for more natural start times.

DO YOU HAVE A SLEEP DISORDER?

Sleep disorders are very common. Sometimes they are unrelated to other problems, but often they are caused by medication side effects or other medical disorders. Sleep disorders are usually associated with one or more of the following symptoms: very loud snoring, waking up gasping for air, needing to move your legs when you're trying to sleep, excessive moving when you are sleeping, and feeling tired the next day. If you suspect that you may have a sleep disorder, make sure you discuss it with your doctor. If these disorders disrupt your sleep, they can, in turn, disrupt your memory.

SHOULD YOU USE SLEEPING PILLS?

If you're having trouble falling asleep, should you use sleeping pills? Yes and no. There are two "sleeping pills" that are generally safe to use and will not compromise your memory or increase your risk for dementia: *melatonin* and *acetaminophen.*

Melatonin

As we described earlier in this chapter, melatonin is a hormone that your body makes to help regulate your sleep cycle. When levels of melatonin rise, it tells your body to prepare for sleep. If you are having difficulty regulating your sleep cycle for whatever reason—including because you are jet-lagged—you may benefit from taking melatonin. Let your doctor know if you are interested in this medication, as it can interact with other medicines.

But before you reach for that bottle, see if you can make your own melatonin by spending at least 30 minutes outside or near a bright, sunlit window between 1 and 3 p.m. That sun exposure will help you to generate your own melatonin approximately 8 hours later, between 9 and 11 p.m. Many of us, unfortunately, work indoors where we don't have the opportunity to spend time in the sun. And the problem is compounded in the winter when cold temperatures may dissuade you from venturing outside.

For this reason, it may be beneficial to regulate your sleep cycle with melatonin pills, at least for a while until your body gets into a good rhythm. Then you may be able to stop the pills because you've trained your body to follow a good cycle. Start with 0.5 milligrams (mg) 1 hour before your desired sleep time, and increase in the following doses every 2 to 3 weeks until you're sleeping better or you've reached the highest dose: 1, 3, 6, 9, 12, 15 mg. After trying a number of doses, reduce the dose to the lowest one that works equally well. In other words, if you try all the doses up to 15 mg but you find that the 3-mg dose works as well as 15 mg, reduce the dose to 3 mg.

Remember that melatonin regulates your sleep cycle and does not make you instantaneously fall asleep, so NEVER take melatonin in the middle of the night or you may prevent yourself from going to sleep at a normal time.

Acetaminophen

Are you ever kept up at night by joint aches, back pains, sore muscles, or a stiff neck? Many people are. It is for this reason that acetaminophen (also known as paracetamol, brand names Tylenol, Panadol, and many others), a mild pain reliever, can help you to fall asleep. As always, let your doctor know if you want to try this approach. We recommend taking a single 325 mg-pill about 30 minutes before your desired sleep time.

Don't Take Other Prescription or Over-the-Counter Sleeping Pills

What about all the other prescription and over-the-counter sleeping pills out there? We strongly urge you not to take them.

Sleeping pills do not produce natural sleep. They sedate you. They impair your episodic and procedural memory, not only for information and skills you learned earlier that day, but also for information and skills you're trying to learn the next day. Many also cause dependence, such that it is harder to fall asleep without them. A large meta-analysis reviewing the data in about 4,500 people found that sleeping pills produced only "slight improvements," averaging 22 minutes, in the speed of falling asleep compared to placebo pills.[16]

Our strong recommendation—supported by the American College of Physicians—is not to take sleeping pills (other than melatonin and acetaminophen) if you want to optimize your memory. Twenty-two minutes to fall asleep faster is negligible compared to the impairment of memory that these sleeping pills cause. Few people fall asleep the moment their head hits the pillow. There is nothing wrong with settling down in bed for 10 to 20 minutes before you fall asleep.

So what should you do instead of taking pills if you're having more trouble falling asleep? Use nonpharmacological techniques to help your sleep as described at the end of this chapter, or ask your doctor about referring you for cognitive behavioral therapy.

Are you thinking of using alcohol to help you sleep? Alcohol actually disrupts and fragments sleep, interfering with the beneficial properties of sleep—in addition to interfering with learning and memory, as discussed in Chapter 19.

DON'T CRAM: STUDY, SLEEP, REPEAT

Let's now return to our story at the beginning of this chapter. Entering college, you took two new languages. Although you devoted equal time for each, for Arabic you studied for 1 hour each day, 4 days a week, for 10 weeks totaling 40 hours. For German you studied 10 hours a day for the 2 days prior to the midterm and the 2 days prior to the final, also totaling

40 hours. You received straight A's in both classes. But returning to school the next year, you found that you retained one of the languages quite well, while the other had almost completely vanished. By this point in the chapter, you should know which language was retained, which vanished, and why.

By studying Arabic 1 hour each day—and then sleeping on that information—you didn't overload your hippocampus with information, and there was time for the information stored in your hippocampus each day to be consolidated each night, forming new and long-lasting episodic and semantic memories. So, not only could you remember Arabic for your exams, you were also able to retain the information for the next year.

By contrast, when you crammed your German studying into 10 hours a day over just 4 days, your hippocampus was simply unable to transfer all of the information it learned to your cortex in just a few night's sleep. This is one of the main reasons that you should space out your learning and not cram for tests.

SLEEP TO REMEMBER

Here are some tips to enhance sleep and optimize your memory.[17]

- Review material you wish to remember shortly before bed. This reduces interference from other information and will increase the likelihood the information is strengthened in memory overnight.
- If you listen to calm, relaxing music while you are studying, try listening to the same music while you are getting ready for sleep. This may increase the likelihood that the information you studied is reactivated overnight.
- Don't cram. Space out your learning. Remember: Study, sleep, repeat.
- Don't pull an all-nighter; you'll remember more information if you give yourself time to sleep.
- Make sure you get enough sleep each night.

- Remember that you likely need between 7 and 9 hours in bed trying to sleep each night to get your required amount of sleep. Start with 8 hours in bed if you're not sure what's right for you and give yourself more time if you need it (or less if you need less time).
- How do you know if you are getting enough sleep each night? Ask yourself the following questions. If you answered "no" to one or more of these, try giving yourself more time to sleep and see if you feel better.
  - Would you wake up close to the time of your alarm clock even if you forgot to set it?
  - Are you feeling rested and not sleepy in the late morning?
  - Can you function optimally without caffeine before noon?
  - Can you attend a boring lecture or movie with the lights out without struggling to stay awake?
- What if you have insomnia, trouble falling asleep? Or waking up in the middle of the night?
  - When you get up in the morning, do you feel well rested? Are you awake and alert throughout the day? Can you answer "yes" to all of the preceding questions regarding how you know if you are getting enough sleep each night? If so, you may simply not need to be in bed for as long as you are giving yourself. Try shortening your time in bed by 15 minutes each week until you find you can go to sleep more quickly or you've reached a minimum of 7 hours.
  - Remember that it's normal for many people to spend 15 to 20 minutes in bed before falling sleep; you shouldn't consider that a problem.
  - Recall also that during normal sleep there are several brief awakenings during the night; if you can return to sleep in 10 to 15 minutes (perhaps after using the toilet) this isn't generally a problem.
  - Stimulate your own melatonin release by being exposed to sunlight first thing in the morning and for at least 30 minutes each day in the early afternoon (usually 1 to 3 p.m. is best).
  - **Go to bed and wake up at the same time each day—weekends the same as weekdays.** This is so important we had to make it bold. If you need to ease into this, first set a standard wake time.

After doing this for a couple of weeks, you will likely find that you start to feel tired around the same time each night. Listen to your body and use that as your standard bedtime.

o If you nap, it should not be after 3 p.m. or for more than 20 to 30 minutes. (If you nap for longer you are likely to wake during deep sleep—which will lead you to feel sluggish for quite a while—and it may be difficult to fall asleep at night.)

o Use a comfortable mattress and pillow.

o Bedrooms should be gadget-free (no beeps or lights), dark, and cool (generally between 65 and 68 degrees Fahrenheit [18 to 20 degrees Celsius]).

o If you watch the clock trying to fall asleep or return to sleep, turn it around or remove it.

o Don't look at blue LED screens (such as on computers, tablets, and smartphones) prior to or in bed. Even with blue-light filters on, screen time in the hour before bed can work against a good night's sleep.

o Don't look at emails or do other non-relaxing activities as you are going to bed.

o Reduce anxiety and worry before getting into bed. Read a book, listen to music, practice meditation, or take a hot bath. Try to establish a nightly routine that helps your body know it is time for sleep.

o Exercise during the day; this will help you fall asleep and sleep soundly at night. (Note: Exercise in the evenings or night can keep you awake.)

o Caffeinated beverages (such as coffee, tea, colas, and energy drinks) can keep you awake, so make sure you have them early in the day, perhaps just in the morning. Quantity matters as well. You may do best without any caffeinated beverages. Remember that "decaffeinated" coffee still has some caffeine it—you may need to cut that out as well, particularly in the afternoon or evening. Chocolate (including hot chocolate) contains a caffeine-like substance and can also keep you awake.

o Don't use nicotine. It is also a stimulant and can keep you awake.

o Reduce your alcohol consumption, particularly in the evening and night. Although it may seem like alcohol helps sleep, it does not. Alcohol fragments sleep and causes many brief unremembered awakenings. It also suppresses REM sleep, which is why hallucinations are one symptom of alcohol withdrawal. The hallucinations may actually be REM sleep rebounding and breaking into waking consciousness.

- Avoid large meals and beverages late at night. Fruit, although healthy, contains lots of water and may require your needing to use the toilet in the middle of the night.
- Some prescription medications that can be taken at any time of day will disrupt your sleep if you take them at night. Ask your doctor about whether it is safe to move some of your nighttime medications to the afternoon or morning.
- If you have been lying in bed for 30 minutes and are getting anxious about falling asleep or are feeling activated, get up and do something quiet and relaxing in a different quiet and dimly lit room until you feel calmer.
- If you have been lying in bed for 30 minutes and are not feeling anxious or activated, but are just relaxing and dozing, then you may not need to get out of bed. Dozing, relaxing, and daydreaming in bed with your eyes closed can have restorative value as long as it is during your usual sleeping time.
- If you're still having trouble falling asleep, try recording a sleep log for at least 2 weeks. Track what time you get into bed, what time you try to fall asleep, what time you get up, how rested (or not) you feel, how many times you recall being up in the night (and for approximately how long), how many caffeinated beverages you consume during the day and at what time, how much exercise you do and at what times, the times and foods you have at your meals, and other information you think may be important. Compare your log with the information you learned in this chapter. You'll likely see many ways you can improve your sleep.
- Lastly, it is completely normal to have trouble sleeping a couple of times each month. That isn't a sign that something is wrong or that you need to change your sleep habits.

21

Activity, attitude, music, mindfulness, and brain training

You look through the window at the beautiful day outside. People are walking, children are playing, but you are inside sitting at your computer. Your phone rings and you answer it. "No," you respond, "I'm sorry, I can't go for a walk with you today, I need to work on this computerized brain-training program . . . You're going dancing later? Hmm . . . that sounds like fun, but I should probably do another of these computer modules." You finish the call, sigh, pull your eyes away from the window, and return to the computer program.

Are computerized brain-training programs the best way to keep your memory strong and your brain healthy, or it is better to walk and dance with friends? Are there benefits to listening to music, or is it just a pleasant distraction? Is there anything to that mindfulness meditation stuff? How important is it to have a positive attitude? We'll answer these questions and more in this chapter.

PARTICIPATE IN SOCIAL ACTIVITIES

We Are Social Animals

The human brain did not evolve to solve crossword or Sudoku puzzles. Humans are social animals and, in part, our brain evolved to understand and facilitate complex social interactions.[1] If we needed a reminder regarding the importance of social activities for our cognitive and emotional health, the COVID-19 pandemic provided one. The social isolation necessitated by the pandemic and the resulting loneliness and disconnection you may have experienced put not only your emotional health at risk, but your cognitive health as well.

Social Engagement and Cognitive Impairment

If you are middle-aged or older, engaging in social activities has been shown to reduce your risk of cognitive decline and the subsequent development of mild cognitive impairment and dementia.[2] These effects are not small; one group of researchers from Rush University in Chicago followed over 1,000 older adults for 5 years and found that those individuals who were the most socially active showed 70% less cognitive decline compared to those with the lowest rates of social activities.[3] (It should be noted, however, that these risk reductions are usually based upon correlations, meaning that it is also possible that what some of these studies are really telling us is that those who are beginning to develop cognitive impairment stop participating in social activities.)

Seek Positive Social Interactions

Not surprisingly, beneficial social interactions for cognitive health are those described as "positive" and "enjoyable." Negative social interactions can put you at risk for cognitive decline.[4] So, whatever your age, we recommend that you seek out and cultivate positive social interactions. Don't forget that in addition to school, work, and your existing network of friends and family, you can consider becoming active in a local community center, club, or lodge. There are many social activities associated with religious organizations at mosques, synagogues, churches, and other meeting houses. You can also socialize by joining a class to learn a new sport, hobby, language, or game. There are many opportunities to be socially engaged, so choose one today and improve your brain health!

LISTEN TO MUSIC

Music Turns on the Brain

After social activities, there is probably nothing that activates as many parts of your brain as listening to music. Music can synchronize the activity of many brain regions, including your auditory cortex processing sound, your visual cortex processing vision, and your prefrontal cortex coordinating your brain activity—perhaps best described as the "conductor" of your brain's orchestra in this discussion.[5] Music also activates your brain's motor system involved in movement, including some of the same regions involved in procedural memory: premotor cortex and cerebellum (the little brain). These connections to your motor system are theorized to allow you to pick out the beat of the music.[6] Lastly, music activates your emotional and episodic memory regions as well, including those next to the hippocampus.[7]

Music Makes You Feel Good

Perhaps because of the positive feelings it can engender, people associate music with a variety of beneficial aspects of emotional health and cognitive function. The AARP (formerly the American Association of Retired Persons) surveyed over 3,000 adults aged 18 and older and found that music was associated with self-reported reduced levels of anxiety and depression, very good or excellent brain health, good quality of life, happiness and mental well-being, and the ability to learn new things.[8]

Music Therapy and Dancing Benefit Older Adults

Music therapy has been successfully used to improve mood and memory in individuals with mild or moderate Alzheimer's disease dementia. M. Gómez Gallego and J. Gómez García, researchers in Murcia, Spain, found that 12 sessions of music therapy improved patients' overall cognitive function on the Mini-Mental State Examination (better known as the MMSE) from 15.0 to 19.6 out of a possible 30 points—that's the equivalent of turning the clock back on this disease by almost 2 years.[9] Music has also been shown to positively engage preserved old memories in individuals with moderate to severe dementia, turning otherwise withdrawn and sedentary individuals into lively, dancing ones.[10]

In fact, by combining music with exercise and social interaction, dancing has been found to be particularly beneficial in healthy older adults. A meta-analysis found that dance interventions from 10 weeks to 18 months either maintained or improved cognitive performance.[11]

Study to the Right Tunes

Should you study with music? Will it help, hurt, or have no effect on your memory? Different investigators have found different results. However, Claudia Echaide, David del Río, and colleagues in Madrid, Spain, may have an explanation for the divergent findings. They discovered that listening to instrumental background music did not affect memory immediately or 48 hours later for a list of unrelated words, but it did impair memory for visuospatial information.[12] The authors interpreted their findings as related to the instrumental music competing in the brain with right-hemisphere visual information but not with left-hemisphere verbal information. If the authors are correct and you're listening to songs with lots of words, it might interfere with your studying for your vocabulary test, while instrumental music might impair your studying for your art history final.

Music also may motivate you to lengthen your study sessions and to persevere longer in your attempts to understand new material. You may stay in the library longer (away from the temptations of social media) if your studying is accompanied by a soundtrack you like. The positive mood evoked by the music may also help to offset stress that you're feeling about an upcoming exam—stress that might otherwise disrupt your ability to understand and learn material.

So, listen to music that you like when you study—but don't let it compete with the material you are trying to learn.

Dance the Night Away

Whether you are young or old, our recommendations are to listen to music that you enjoy. Even better, move with the music, whether that means swaying in your bedroom to soft jazz, jumping in your living room to hip hop, or dancing the night away to disco.

TRAIN YOUR BRAIN: PRACTICE MINDFULNESS

Don't Forget to Pay Attention

Paying attention is the first step in remembering information, including where you parked your car, the talking points in your sales pitch, or the name of the woman who just introduced herself. Paying attention is a deceptively simple concept but, as discussed in Parts 1 and 2, it is not always easy to accomplish. We are all easily distracted. You may be thinking about the errands you need to complete at the mall and not where you are parking in the garage. You may be so nervous about the sales pitch you have to give in the morning that you can't concentrate on the talking points you're supposed to memorize. Perhaps the appetizers going by look so enticing that you're not paying any attention to the woman as she's telling you her name. Because you weren't paying attention, it is no surprise that you cannot recall where you parked, your talking points, or the woman's name.

Improve Attention by Practicing Mindfulness

One way to improve your ability to pay attention—and therefore improve your memory—is to practice mindfulness. Mindfulness training can teach you how to be present in the moment and pay attention to whatever you are doing. Many studies have shown that practicing mindfulness can improve your ability to pay attention and remember.[13,14]

How does mindfulness training improve attention? Ben Isbel, Mathew Summers, and their colleagues at the University of the Sunshine Coast, Australia, performed an intriguing experiment in an attempt to answer this question. They examined the changes in the electrical activity of the brain as detected by an electroencephalogram (better known as an EEG) in healthy older adults who spent 6 months engaged in mindfulness training. The training involved asking participants to cultivate mindful awareness of the sensations accompanying the breath. In addition to performing significantly better on a task measuring attention, the researchers observed EEG changes that suggested two different brain processes were enhanced. Mindfulness training increased the efficiency of brain pathways that process incoming information coming up from the senses, and it also boosted the ability of the brain's central executive to direct attention down to the information of interest. Thus, mindfulness training enhanced both the "bottom up" and "top down" processes that facilitate attention, as described in Chapter 3.[15]

Start with 1 Minute

Although practicing mindfulness isn't for everyone, it might be right for you. If you'd like to give it a try, there are many ways to learn how to do it. In addition to virtual and in-person classes, there are also print and audio books, online videos, and smartphone applications that can get you started. Andrew spends a dozen minutes each morning being mindful. Elizabeth practices mindfulness as well. We both recommend that you find a time that you can integrate mindfulness into your daily routine, such as when you first wake up, as part of your bedtime routine, or perhaps as you're cooling down from exercising. We also recommend starting small—perhaps just 1 minute each day—and increasing by 1 minute each week until you reach your target. After you've mastered the basics of focusing on your breath, you may be able to incorporate mindfulness into other activities, such as walking from your car to your office.

HAVE A POSITIVE ATTITUDE

Can a positive attitude really make a difference? The short answer is yes, it can make all the difference in the world. A positive attitude can sustain your memory—and your brain—over time. On the other hand, a negative attitude can actually impair your memory. Let's look at a couple of the reasons why.

Attitude and Behavior

Becca Levy and her colleagues at Yale University conducted several studies that have examined the long-term effects of attitude on memory in older adults. Looking at 38 years of data from the Baltimore Longitudinal Study of Aging, she found that older adults who held more positive views about aging (such as "With age comes wisdom") showed 30% less decline in their memory compared with those who held more negative views (such as "Old people are absent-minded").[16]

How is this possible? The answer is likely related to another study she and her colleagues conducted examining the self-perceptions of 241 older individuals who participated in the Ohio Longitudinal Study of Aging and Retirement. Here she discovered that those with more positive attitudes tended to practice more preventive health behaviors, like engaging in regular exercise, eating a balanced diet, and taking their medications as prescribed.[17] So, one reason that attitude makes such a difference for memory and brain health is that a positive attitude can produce positive behaviors.

A Self-Fulfilling Prophecy

Attitude can also have more immediate effects. Memory performance can be altered in mere minutes by giving people words or statements that are related to a stereotype that is threatening to them. For example, older adults perform worse on tests of memory when shown negative words about aging such as "decrepit" and "senile," compared to when they are shown positive words such as "wise" and "sage." These effects can even come out accidentally at a doctor's office if the implication is, now that you're older, it's expected that your memory will be impaired.[18]

Don't Have a Positive Attitude? Change It!

Although there is ongoing research to understand exactly how these threatening stereotypes affect one's memory and other abilities, two things are clear. First, while these effects are small, they are also very real and have been replicated in dozens of studies. Second, there are many ways to reduce, eliminate, or even reverse these stereotype effects. For example, although Black students performed poorly on a verbal test when told that it was "diagnostic" of their verbal abilities, their performance improved dramatically simply by the test being described as "non-diagnostic" of their verbal abilities—therefore removing the threat that poor performance could confirm a negative stereotype.[19] And we already mentioned that older adults perform better on tests of memory when shown positive words about aging.

The bottom line is that, while it might sound like pseudo-science or mere "pop psychology," attitude really does make a difference. So, if you don't have a positive attitude, work on changing it today!

ENGAGE IN NOVEL, MENTALLY STIMULATING ACTIVITIES

Researchers from the Mayo Clinic in Rochester, Minnesota, followed 2,000 healthy adults aged 70 years and older for 5 years, looking to see what factors would protect them from memory loss and mild cognitive impairment (see Chapter 13). They found that engaging in two, three, four, or five mentally stimulating activities in late life correlated with a lower risk for developing memory loss, with a trend suggesting that the more activities, the lower the risk. Some of the reported beneficial activities in both midlife and late life included social activities, computer use, and board games. Crafts were also beneficial in late life.[20] Activities that have shown benefits from other studies include playing musical instruments and dancing.

Seek Novelty

Even more impressive are the benefits seen when individuals engage in a novel activity, such as learning a new skill, taking up a new hobby, or visiting a new place. In fact, a group of researchers from Case Western Reserve University in Ohio observed the lowest risk of developing Alzheimer's disease in individuals who most frequently participated in novelty-seeking activities.[21]

Can older adults improve their thinking and memory abilities by training on novel, mentally stimulating activities? This was the question that Lesley Tranter and Wilma Koutstaal, psychologists at the University of Reading, England, set out to answer. They found that after 10 to 12 weeks of training on novel, mentally stimulating activities, measures of problem-solving and flexible thinking increased significantly.[22]

Minimize Television and Social Media

If novel, mentally stimulating activities are helpful, you might wonder whether there are other types of activities that could be bad for your brain. The answer is "yes." In one study, Heather Lindstrom and colleagues at Case Western Reserve University used questionnaires gathered from 135 individuals with Alzheimer's disease and 331 healthy older adults to examine the number of hours spent on 26 leisure activities when they were between 40 and 59 years old. After controlling for year of birth, gender, income, and education, they found that each additional daily hour of watching television in midlife increased the risk of Alzheimer's disease in late life 1.3 times. By contrast, participating in intellectually stimulating activities and social activities reduced the risk of developing Alzheimer's.[23] Other studies suggest that high levels of social media use can similarly be associated with increased memory failures. Interestingly, some of the effects of social media seem to be linked to their tendency to increase negative emotions, working against your attempts to maintain a positive outlook.[24] So, turn off the tube, stop scrolling through online posts, and use that time to engage in more mentally stimulating activities that may help both your mood and your memory.

Find Stimulating Activities in Your Daily Life

Putting all this data together, the message is clear. Whether you are young, middle-aged, or in your golden years, it's best to engage in novel, mentally stimulating activities. Such activities most certainly include social activities, but they also include learning new skills and hobbies and visiting new places. If you are in school, that is a wonderful place to engage in novel, mentally stimulating activities of all types—including your coursework. If you are working at a job that provides such stimulation, that's great as well. If, however, you are retired or your job does not provide the right type of stimulation, we recommend that you find hobbies, sports, or other activities that do.

WHAT ABOUT COMPUTERIZED BRAIN-TRAINING GAMES?

Watch Out for Exaggerated Claims

If novel, mentally stimulating activities are beneficial, what about all of those computerized brain-training games out there: Are they beneficial? The companies who make these games would like you to think so. Unfortunately, these companies often make exaggerated claims—so much so that in 2015 and 2016 the U.S. Federal Trade Commission imposed fines and ordered the removal of unsubstantiated claims from the products' advertising materials.[25,26]

Do Some Computerized Brain-Training Programs Work?

OK, so some products exaggerate their benefits. But are other products worthwhile? It's a complicated question, in part because there are hundreds of brain-training programs out there (with more being added every day), and in part because the right studies with proper controls are rarely conduced. When the proper controls are done, the results are generally negative.

For example, a group of researchers at the Icahn School of Medicine at Mount Sinai, in New York City, examined the effectiveness of a marketed computerized cognitive training program in adults aged 80 years and older. Importantly, they compared the training program to an active control of playing computer games that would maintain participants' interest but was not designed to improve their cognition. The results showed that neither group improved their thinking and memory and there were no differences between the groups at the end of the study.[27]

Some studies have shown positive effects. Researchers at the University of Iowa examined whether a group of older adults would benefit from computerized cognitive training compared to an active control group who performed casual computer games. At the end of 10 weeks, the cognitive training group showed greater improvements in the speed by which they were able to process information and their working memory—their ability to hold information in mind and manipulate it (see Chapter 3).[28]

Do It If You Enjoy It

How do we reconcile these and dozens of similar pairs of results that disagree with one another? We agree with the comments of a group of scientists from both the United States and the United Kingdom who also grappled with this issue. They concluded that when individuals participate in computerized brain-training programs there is good evidence that participants get better at the specific tasks that are trained by the program, less evidence that participants improve their performance on similar tasks, and very little evidence that they improve their cognitive performance in daily life activities.[29]

So, if you purchased a computerized brain-training program and you are enjoying it—that's wonderful. We recommend you consider it a hobby, something you do to have fun, rather than something critically important for your brain. Similarly, if you enjoy solving crossword or Sudoku puzzles, by all means continue, but understand that these activities—while much better than television—are not as good as the other activities mentioned in this chapter, such as social activities or engaging in novel, mentally stimulating activities.

HOW TO KEEP YOUR MEMORY STRONG AND YOUR BRAIN HEALTHY

In addition to performing regular aerobic exercise, eating Mediterranean-style meals, limiting alcohol and cannabis, not using illegal drugs, and sleeping well, the following activities we just reviewed will help to keep your memory strong:

- Participate in social activities.
- Listen to music.
  - Likely because it combines exercise, social activities, and music, dancing may be one of the best activities to keep your memory strong.
- Practice mindfulness.
  - Mindfulness can improve your ability to focus your attention, which, in turn, will help you remember.
- Keep a positive mental attitude.
- Engage in novel, cognitively stimulating activities.

But what about if you want to improve your ability to remember something specific, such as people's names, mathematical formulas, or vocabulary words? To accomplish these feats of memory we now turn to Part 5, where we will show you how to use memory strategies, aids, and mnemonics.

Part 5

TECHNIQUES
TO REMEMBER BETTER

22

Memory aids

"Now what are the things I need to get?" you ask yourself as you're standing in the supermarket aisle. "I think it was almond milk, olive oil, plain yogurt, strawberries, blueberries, soybeans, and sunflower seeds . . . unless it was soy milk, sunflower oil, strawberry and blueberry yogurt, string beans, and almonds?" You sigh and look at your watch, wondering if anyone will be at home that you can call to check on what you were supposed to get. Noticing the time, you slap your forehead, exclaiming, "Oh no! I forgot to take my antibiotic."

Throughout this book we have provided insights that can help you improve your memory based on hundreds of published scientific studies as well as our educational and clinical experience. Our goals in Chapter 22 and the rest of Part 5 are to compile this information scattered throughout the book into one place and to describe additional strategies and aids that can help you remember just about anything—including your grocery list and your medications as in our little story above. Note that if you've just jumped to Part 5 and you haven't read the chapters in Part 4, please review at least the bullets at the end of each chapter, as exercise, nutrition, sleep, social activities, attitude, limiting alcohol/cannabis/drugs, and the other issues discussed there are critically important for memory.

The content of Part 5 comes from many sources. In addition to those we have listed in the earlier chapters of this book, we also incorporated information from *Make It Stick: The Science of Successful Learning*, by Peter C. Brown, Henry L. Roediger III, and Mark A. McDaniel,[1] *Ageless Memory: The Memory Expert's Prescription for a Razor-Sharp Mind*, by Harry Lorayne,[2] and *Moonwalking with Einstein: The Art and Science of Remembering Everything*, by Joshua Foer,[3] in addition to Andrew's earlier book with Maureen K. O'Connor, *Seven Steps to Managing Your Memory: What's Normal, What's Not, and What to Do About It.*[4]

USE MEMORY AIDS

Whether you are young or old, in school or working, or think you have a good or bad memory, you can use external memory aids—physical devices, software programs, or phone apps—to help you remember information. Why memorize your shopping list when you can write it down? Why keep appointments in your head when you can keep them in a calendar or your phone? This advice of course assumes that you will have the memory aid with you at the relevant times; if there's a good chance you won't (perhaps you'll need to use a password when not by your computer that contains your password manager), then you'll want to supplement your use of memory aids with the strategies we discuss in later chapters.

Some people worry that their memory will wither away if they use memory aids to improve their memory. We would argue that there are enough things in life that you really do need to memorize, such that if an external memory aid can help, you should take advantage of it. Or, if you're determined to work at memorizing all information (and good for you), you can always memorize that list *and* use an external memory aid—just to double-check you remembered everything correctly.

FIVE GENERAL PRINCIPLES

There are five general principles that will help you use memory aids most effectively.

1. *Be organized.* Use a system so that you know which aid you will use to remember which piece of information.
2. *Be ready.* Whether you use a pencil-and-paper notebook or your phone, be ready to use your external memory aid whenever needed.
3. *Don't delay.* Enter appointments immediately in your paper, phone, or computer calendar. When a reminder pops up to alert you, take care of it right away.
4. *Keep it simple.* Use the simplest memory aid that can accomplish the task. Don't use a complicated system of reminder notes when a daily planner will do. There's no need to purchase a deluxe phone app if a simple app will get the job done.
5. *Develop routines.* The first few times that you use new memory aids it may take a bit of extra thought or effort. But once you get into the routine, they will become part of your procedural memory and easy to use even if you are feeling distracted, rushed, or tired.

SPECIAL PLACES

Benjamin Franklin liked to say, "A place for everything and everything in its place." This is good advice. We've used the example in this book of why you might forget where you put your keys and how you can better remember where you put them. But the best solution is to always put them in the same place every day—that way you never need to look for them. Do the same for your wallet, phone, rings, glasses, and everything else you use daily.

What to do if you don't have a special place for these items? It's the perfect time to create one. Some potential good places are:

- On a table, tray, or bowl near the door where you enter your home, or perhaps on your kitchen table.

- In a small basket that uses suction or magnets to stick to your refrigerator.
- In a tray or bowl on your bedroom dresser or bedside table.
- On top of or in a drawer of your home office desk.
- In your briefcase, purse, or commuter bag.

Which place is best for you will depend, in part, on where you tend to use these items. For example, you might keep your glasses and headphones in your briefcase or purse, and your keys, wallet, and rings in the bedroom. Other factors to consider include how likely it is that your home might be broken into—if it is likely, you'll want to keep expensive items out of sight (perhaps in a drawer) rather than in the open by the door.

CALENDARS AND PLANNERS

Most people use a calendar or daily planner, but not everyone takes full advantage of them. Some people prefer physical, paper planners, although most people today use phone- or web-based calendars. Whichever type you use, make sure that you include the five "W"s in each appointment: *who, what* times 2, *when,* and *where.*

- *Who* is the appointment with?
- *What* is the appointment for?
- *What* should you bring with you or have prepared for the meeting?
- *When* is the appointment?
- *Where* is the appointment located?

Make sure you include the physical or web-based virtual meeting room address. We suggest you also include a backup phone number and/or email address just in case you run into trouble finding the physical or virtual location.

We recommend that you keep your calendar with you so that you can always add appointments as they arise. Whatever type of calendar you use, it's good to periodically create a backup copy just in case it gets lost. Most electronic calendars have built-in backups, and you might want to make copies (perhaps take pictures with your phone) of paper calendars.

TO-DO LISTS

To-do lists can vary from a simple, single list on paper to web- and app-based four-quadrant project-management systems. We recommend matching the complexity of the list to the task.

Simple Lists

If you're going to the supermarket there is nothing wrong with a pen-and-paper list that you can have handy when you're going up and down the aisles. These types of simple lists also work great for other shopping lists, errands, holiday lists, and more.

The Four-Quadrant System

Dwight D. Eisenhower noted, "I have two kinds of problems, the urgent and the important. The urgent are not important, and the important are never urgent."[5] Based on recognizing this critical difference between importance and urgency, we recommend you use what is often called the four-quadrant time-management system or the Eisenhower method when making lists for work, school, or other projects.

Important/Urgent	Important/Not Urgent
Crises you should attend to first	Long-range projects you need to remember
Not Important/Urgent	**Not Important/Not Urgent**
Interruptions, but things you may need to do	Timewasters you should likely avoid altogether

This method has the benefit of allowing you to remember what is important, even if it isn't urgent. It also allows you to see what you should do first, and what you should not bother doing. We recommend that you use a separate paper-, app-, or web-based grid like this for each area of your life (work, school, personal), school subject (history, mathematics, science), or large work project (different ventures or clients, etc.).

REMINDERS

Whether paper sticky notes or electronic pop-ups and alarms, everyone can benefit from reminders of medications, meetings, appointments, projects, and deadlines. App- and web-based systems usually have built-in reminders—don't forget that you can customize them if you wish, so that you're reminded of a meeting 5 minutes ahead of time instead of 15 if that's what you prefer. If you use sticky notes, make sure that you put them somewhere that you'll see them (such as the bathroom mirror or front door) and take them down once you've used them.

PILLBOXES

Medications are important, and serious consequences can result if they are missed or taken twice. Why rely on your memory to determine if you've taken your medication when a pillbox can do it for you? Even with just one or two medications to take, many people have a brief lapse of attention or a false memory (see Chapter 12) and end up missing their medication or taking it twice by accident. Don't let that happen to you.

There are many different pillbox styles available. The basic pillbox has one compartment for each day of the week, and comes in 1-week, 2-week, and 4-week options. There are also two-compartment boxes for morning and evening medications, and three-compartment options for morning, afternoon, and evening medications. If you have afternoon medications, you might also want a pocket-size pillbox that you can take with you when you're out and about.

Some pillboxes have built-in reminder alarms, display screens, and even communication devices that alert family members if medications are being forgotten. Lastly, many pharmacies will prepare your medications in daily, plastic "blister packs" for you either free or for a small charge. Talk to your doctor if you're not sure what the right pillbox is for you.

MEMORY AIDS CAN HELP

Our recommendation is to always consider using a memory aid to remember information if it is important and/or easy to do so.

- Five general principles to use memory aids effectively: *Be organized. Be ready. Don't delay. Keep it simple. Develop routines.*
- A place for everything and everything in its place.
- Include the 5 *W*'s in your calendar or planner: *Who, What* is it for, *What* do you need, *When,* and *Where.*
- Use simple lists for simple tasks.
- Use the four-quadrant system for projects: *important/urgent, important/not urgent, not important/urgent, not important/not urgent.*
- Use reminders.
- Use a pillbox.

23

Basic strategies

You read the textbook chapter and highlighted the key points. Then you re-read the chapter several times. It felt easier each time you read through it such that, by the last read, you were completely confident that you mastered the content. Yet—to your dismay—now you find yourself struggling on the test! You know you read the relevant material, but you just can't remember it.

Would you like to learn the best ways to study—and avoid the studying techniques that give you the illusion of mastery without the knowledge? Do you need to remember your shopping list, appointments for the day, mathematical formulas, anatomical terms, or your company's strategic plan? In this chapter we'll review how to learn whatever content you're trying to remember so that you can breeze through the supermarket, ace your math test, treat your patients correctly, get that promotion, and more.

STRATEGIES WHEN ACQUIRING MEMORIES

Be Motivated
Your ability to remember begins with your desire to remember. If someone is talking and you are not interested in listening

to them, you are unlikely to remember what they are saying—whether they are a colleague introducing themselves or a professor at the podium. So, if you want to remember what someone is saying later, it is important to keep in mind the goals that motivate you to remember what they are saying. This colleague could be a wonderful collaborator on a future project—and you don't want to embarrass yourself and forget their name at the next meeting. And, yes, what the professor is saying may be important not only so you can pass the test but for your later career as well. This principle of motivation is key to all forms of intentional memory. For example, if you want to be able to find your car after the concert, you should be motivated to pay attention to where it is as you are walking away from it in the parking lot.

Align Your In-the-Moment Goals with Your Memory Goals

How many times have you wished you paid more attention at the time when you are later trying to remember information—such as your temporary locker combination or where you left your keys? Being motivated "in theory" isn't enough; if you later want to be able to get into your locker or locate your keys, you have to align your in-the-moment goal when the memory is being formed with your later goal of remembering. So, before you walk away from your locker, take a minute to store the locker number and its combination in your memory. Similarly, focus on where you are putting your keys as they are leaving your hand. The techniques described later in this chapter and the next two will help you to form and store these memories.

By adjusting your goals, you can also change what you remember from an event. For example, if you go to a party to have fun and enjoy yourself, you'll probably remember the games, smiles, and laughs that you were part of. If you go to the same party to network with people who might be able to help you with your career, you're likely to remember the few individuals who fit that role. And if you're looking for a new style that will best reflect your distinct personality, you will likely remember many of the clothes, haircuts, mannerisms, and speech patterns that you encountered. In each of these situations you may not have been consciously trying to remember. But you were paying close attention while playing games, speaking with individuals who might help your career, and looking for style elements, leading you to remember those aspects of the party.

Relax! Don't Be Anxious

Anxiety can be a source of distraction—particularly if it is making you ruminate on past memory failures or other unpleasant thoughts rather than focusing your attention on the present. There are several things that you can do to reduce your anxiety. For example, it may be helpful to try regularly engaging deep breathing or mindfulness meditation (see Chapter 21).

Sometimes reframing your goals can reduce your anxiety. For example, if you believe that you are bad at remembering people's names, and you're meeting someone new right now, having a motivating goal of "remembering their name" may only serve to heighten your anxiety. A more targeted, less intimidating goal such as, "I'm going to form a visual image to help me remember their name," may help you to feel less anxious and remember the name better. Similarly, if you're anxious that you have five chapters of reading or 25 slides to prepare and memorize, try focusing on just one chapter or one slide— something that doesn't sound too intimidating. Once you've finished one chapter or slide, move on to the next. Usually, once you get started, you'll find your stress levels are back to normal.

Use Effort to Do FOUR Things

If we only had space to discuss one strategy in this book, using effort would be the one. Nothing will help you to remember information more than using effort. Consciously trying to remember can be a powerful way to bring your efforts into alignment with your goals of retaining information. In fact, if your studying seems too easy, sometimes that means whatever studying technique you are using is not going to be very effective for learning the material. You will succeed when your goals lead you to exert effort toward processing the information.

We recommend that you use effort to do *FOUR* things: *F*ocus your attention; *O*rganize, cluster, and chunk the information; *U*nderstand the material; and *R*elate the new information to things you already know.

Focus Your Attention

A key part of effort is being present and paying attention to whatever activity, event, or material you're trying to remember. Work to focus on what you want to remember and try to ignore everything else. It takes effort to focus your attention but, as we just discussed, using effort will help you remember. Sit up straight in your chair. If you find your attention drifting, direct it back to the material, experience, lecture, or meeting you wish to remember. If you were lost in thought when you put down your keys, you are unlikely to recall where you put them; pause in your thoughts and pay attention as you are putting the keys down. If you don't want to tell the same story to the same person twice, pay close attention to who is with you as you tell the story; focus on their facial expressions and reactions as you tell it. Interested in improving your ability to pay attention? Try practicing mindfulness as we described in Chapter 21.

• *Avoid distraction—don't multitask.* Because paying attention is so important for forming memories, we hope it is obvious that you won't remember information well if you are distracted because your attention is drawn to something else at the same time. The studies show that although many people think they are good at multitasking, they are actually wrong! No one is able to do two things at once anywhere close to as well as they could if they just focused on that one task. So, turn off the television, close down those browser tabs, stop checking your messages, set your phone to "do not disturb"—and then put your phone out of sight. Just having your phone nearby can be a distractor.

- *Take breaks.* If you find that you are getting mentally fatigued when studying and can no longer focus, take a short break. Go for a walk. Chat with a friend. Grab a snack. Do whatever you need to do to recharge your batteries and get ready for some more studying.
- *Consider a cup of coffee (or tea).* It is important to be alert and attentive—not sleepy or bored—when you are trying to learn new information. Sometimes a cup of coffee or tea can help you to be more alert and pay attention better. However, as described in detail in Chapter 20, coffee and tea are not substitutes for getting a good night's sleep.
- *Use your senses.* One beneficial strategy to help you remember almost any type of experience or information is to use your senses. To remember where you put your keys, listen to the sound they make when you put them in the metal bowl. If you're trying to remember words on a page, give them new dimensions. Don't just read about where the car parts are coming from—visualize the various components traveling from different parts of the world, converging in Detroit, and being assembled into an automobile. If you want to remember a day at the beach, smell the sea air. Feel the sand under your toes as you walk down the beach and the wind as it moves the tiny hairs on your forearms. See the colorful plastic pails and shovels full of sand and salt water. Hear your grandchildren's shrieks and laughs over the sound of the surf as waves try to wash their sandcastles away.
- *Create sensational mnemonics.* You can also use your sensations creatively to help you remember information. For example, did you just meet Barbara wearing a bright pink dress? Imagine her name written in bright pink letters to match her dress. You can also use sounds to remember information—for example, "Because I knew just what to do, I parked my car on level two," or "If I want a beautiful rose, I must remember to water it with the hose."

Organize, Cluster, and Chunk

Material that is organized or clustered together in a logical way is easier to remember than information that is random or ordered in a non-useful way. To use an obvious example, you'll have a more difficult time remembering your groceries if they are ordered like this:

- Apples
- Burger rolls
- Corn (canned)
- Dental floss
- Eggs
- Frozen peas
- Green tomatoes
- Honeydew melons
- Ice cream
- Jarlsberg cheese
- Krispy Kreme donuts
- Lima beans (canned)
- Mouthwash
- Napa cabbage

than if they are clustered by category:

- Apples
- Honeydew melons
- Green tomatoes
- Napa cabbage
- Eggs
- Jarlsberg cheese
- Burger rolls
- Krispy Kreme donuts
- Corn (canned)
- Lima beans (canned)
- Frozen peas
- Ice cream

- Dental floss
- Mouthwash

Similarly, if you're reviewing the names of your old high school friends for your upcoming reunion, try to remember them by the different groups or social circles in which you knew them, rather than the order in the yearbook.

You can also impose organization on material by chunking it. Few people can remember long unbroken lists of numbers or letters, such as the credit card number 1350246791181012. But if you break numbers or letters down into "bite-size" chunks you may find patterns that are helpful, such as odd (1 3 5), even (0 2 4 6), odd (7 9 11), even (8 10 12). You can also turn numbers into other information that may be meaningful to you and/or easier to remember. For example, this number could also be remembered as: 1/3/50 (January 3, 1950); 2/4/67 (February 4, 1967); 9/1/1810 (September 1, 1810); and 12 (December). Even turning it into two-digit numbers will make it easier, as eight numbers are easier to remember than 16: 13 50 24 67 91 18 10 12. You can also relate the chunked two-digit numbers into those you are more familiar with, such as basketball scores or perhaps baseball players' jersey numbers. In this way you can picture the eight two-digit numbers of your credit card assigned to eight different ballplayers in the infield and outfield. We'll also describe other ways to remember numbers in Chapter 25.

Understand

It's almost impossible to remember details, events, or experiences if you don't understand them. So, if you're learning something new, make sure that you understand it well. Extract key ideas, build the ideas into a mental model, and connect the model to your prior knowledge. Giving a presentation on the material (or just preparing to) is one way to ensure that you have truly mastered it. If you're living through an experience that you want to remember forever, think about the meaning of what is happening around you, whether it is a special celebration, an election night, or the birth of a child.

- *Build from the foundations up.* Remember that to understand the new material you are learning, you must first understand the prior material as a foundation. You need to crawl before you walk, master arithmetic before algebra, and understand normal physiology before the diseases that affect it. Make sure that you have mastered the basics. Once you have, work to understand how the new knowledge you are learning fits in with your prior knowledge. Reflect upon the key ideas you are learning. Think of different examples. See how these ideas and examples relate to what you already know. Continue the process of comparing and contrasting the new learning to your existing knowledge as your mastery of a topic grows, making associations as you go.
- *Generate content.* One way to use effort to aid your understanding when learning new information is to force yourself to generate the content in your own words. Distill the key points and say them aloud to yourself or to someone else. Follow the Latin proverb *Docendo discimus*, "by teaching, we learn." Remember, when learning is harder, it's stronger and lasts longer.

Relate—Make Associations

Making associations between the new information you are trying to remember and older information you already know is one of the most powerful memory strategies. You can also make other associations as well. For example, if you tend to lose your reading glasses and you're setting them down on your book, try associating the two so you'll remember. You can imagine a book made out of glass, or perhaps imagine the book wearing the glasses. Even verbally stating the association can help you to remember it later. Say aloud, "I'm putting my glasses down on my book."

Trying to learn a new computer program or smartphone application? Think about how the electronic steps might relate to things you're more familiar with, such as moving paper or other physical objects around and manipulating them.

If you're trying to remember an address, try relating the street name to the number. Below are the some of the most common street names in the United States, each paired with a random number from 1 to 100. Let's see how you can make associations to help you remember the numbers that go with them.

- 65 Park Avenue: 65 is the traditional age that being a "senior citizen" begins. You can therefore picture a white-haired senior citizen parking their car in a special "senior" spot next to the park.
- 76 Main Street: You may know the song that starts, "76 trombones led the big parade." And you almost certainly know that the U.S. Declaration of Independence was signed in 1776. So, you can picture 76 trombones parading down Main Street during an Independence Day celebration.
- 25 Oak Street: Since 25 cents is one quarter, try picturing an oak tree, but instead of acorns, there are quarters hanging off it, and each quarter has an image of acorn on it instead of a face.
- 24 Clear Street: Maybe imagine a forest with two dozen pine trees giving way to a clearing with a house made of glass.
- 99 Washington Street: Perhaps picture a 99-year-old George Washington on his horse riding down the street.
- 54 Lake Street: If you know that 54 is considered a perfect score in golf, you can picture yourself hitting 54 golf balls into a lake.

Did you notice that most of the associations we described involve creating images? This wasn't by accident. One of the best ways to make an association that will be remembered is to make a mental image, which brings us to one of the best ways to relate information: *Create visual images.*

Human beings are visual animals. We probably devote more of our brain to processing visual information than we do to processing all other types of information combined. For this reason, one of the best ways to remember information and relate it to other information is to turn it into a mental image. If you've just met a new colleague at work and you happen to discuss that you both enjoy swimming, picture yourself talking to them underwater—still in your work clothes—and that will help you remember that association.

Note that you can use images for both concrete and abstract information that you want to remember. Look again at the examples we used in the last section. In some, we used concrete examples, such as an image of George Washington for Washington Street, and a lake for Lake Street. But in others we took something abstract, such as the number 25 or the word "Clear," and turned it into a visualizable item, such as a quarter or a clearing and a house made of glass.

You can also create images for abstract concepts based upon what the word sounds like if you are learning new vocabulary words in English or a foreign language. For example, to remember that *jentacular* means related to breakfast, you can picture your friend *Jen tacking you* to a *large* glass of orange juice (a glass so large you can barely reach the top of it). (Note that this method can also be helpful for remembering the million passwords we all need to keep track of.)

Did it seem like a lot of effort was involved to just remember that one word? That's great! As you now know, effort is the key to memory, so anything that gets you to use effort will help you to remember. What's that you're saying? It's a rather silly image you made? That's good, too: The more silly and distinctive the image is, the more likely you will remember it.

Take Ownership of Your Learning

If you're studying, we have every confidence that you will succeed at learning the material. Just the fact that you are taking the time to read this chapter to improve your studying skills tells us a lot about you. You are taking ownership of your learn-ing. You want to study smarter, not just harder. You know that when you put in effort, use the techniques we describe, and are persistent, you are forming new connections in your brain that will actually improve your ability to learn the material you're studying. In a very real sense, you are improving your intel-ligence for that subject.

Part of taking ownership of your learning is that you may not be satisfied by simply studying the textbook, your home-work assignments, or a company's prospectus. If these sources are sufficient for you to excel in your course, prepare for your presentation, and achieve your goals, great! But if you find these techniques are not allowing you to master the material as well as you would like or get the grade you're looking for on the exam, you know that means you need to explore additional methods to achieve success. Studying in small groups with your classmates, attending office hours with your professor, or meeting with cli-ents and other stakeholders may all help you to better master the material. If you thought you mastered the material but you're being asked about it from an angle you didn't expect, you may want to seek out additional textbooks, problem-solving books, websites, or colleagues that will give you information (and per-haps practice) from other perspectives. You and your classmates or colleagues might even have fun designing quizzes or job sce-narios for each other that are as clever and devious as you can imagine to help you prepare for the next test or business meeting. Explore other ways to be successful as well.

Make It Distinctive

Distinctive things are memorable. In fact, one reason that visual images are memorable is that, just by their visual nature, they are generally distinctive. But there are many other ways that you can make the information you're trying to remember distinctive.

- *Involve the senses.* As we discussed earlier in this chapter, you can use real or imagined sights, sounds, smells, tastes, and tactile feelings associated with the information to make it more distinctive and thus more memorable.
- *Use humor.* Silly things are distinctive. That's one reason that many of us can remember jokes, cartoons, and silly slogans so well. One way to remember information is to turn it into something silly. Want to remember 1222 Deer Valley Drive? Picture a *deer driving* through a *valley* while waving at a dozen (*12*) startled hunters with .22-caliber guns.
- *Imbue it with emotion.* If you're reading, listening, or watching something you want to remember, try to feel and experience the hope, joy, sadness, fear, relief, calm, or other emotion of the people in the article, feature, story, or video. Don't just read information about a company on their website; think about how it would feel to work at that company or be a client receiving their services. As you're memorizing vocabulary words, imagine yourself performing the action or using the object, and think about how that makes you feel. If you're learning biochemical pathways, think about the diseases that affect people's lives when these pathways go awry, and imagine yourself helping them as a scientist or doctor.
- *Make it important to you.* If you're trying to remember the points made by a speaker at a meeting or a conference, think about how each point could be relevant in your personal or professional life. So, if you want to remember, "Begin with the end in mind," think about a situation in your own life when you didn't do this and you wish that you had. If you're trying to remember your company's 16 regional offices, think about planning a trip to each location and the city-specific activities that you would do there. If you're trying to learn how to use a new smartphone app, imagine a specific scenario in which you'd implement the steps. (For example, "This is the button I'll press to schedule a car to take me to my friend's house. This is where I'll type in his address. Then, I'll watch this map so I know when to grab my coat and wait outside for the driver.")

Acquire Content in the Way You Will Need to Retrieve It

It's always easier to recall information the same way that you learned it. So, if you're going to be interviewing for a job as a bartender and you know it is likely that they're going to name a dozen drinks and ask you how you would make them, you'll want to make sure that you use the drink name as the cue that triggers your memory for the ingredients—not the other way around. Similarly, if you're going to a client meeting and you're expected to know the data or other information inside and out, work on memorizing the material from multiple angles, so that not only can you say "Cleveland" when they ask you where their major supplier is located, but also, "that's where your major supplier is located," when they mention Cleveland.

To prepare for exams, don't just study material the way it is presented in the textbook; think about how your professor is most likely to test you and study the material that way. Not sure how you will be tested? It can only be beneficial to study the material multiple ways, so that however you will be tested, you will be ready. This will also help you when you need to retrieve the material not only on an exam, but in an upper-level elective that builds upon the material or—more importantly—in your career.

Make Acronyms

One tried-and-tested memory technique that has been used to memorize everything from long speeches to anatomical terms is making acronyms. You may have grown up with Roy G. Biv to help you remember the order of the visual light spectrum (red, orange, yellow, green, blue, indigo, violet) or HOMES to recall the Great Lakes (Huron, Ontario, Michigan, Erie, Superior). You can also create acronyms to help you remember your shopping list (BREAD: bread, rice, eggs, apples, dental floss), your errands (SHOP: shoemaker, hardware store, optician, pet shop), and anything else you would like to remember. Note that acronyms don't have to be pretty; you can use SHoPP for shoe-maker, hardware store, pet shop, podiatrist where the "o" has no referent and there are two P's. The important thing is just that it serves you as a memory aid.

CHOOSE WHETHER YOU WILL REMEMBER OR FORGET IT

Remember that you have some control over what you will later remember and what you will forget. If you want to remember something that you just heard or saw, think to yourself, "I want to remember this information so I can tell my friend about it later," or for whatever the reason is. That simple thought will help you remember it—and you might also want to use some of the other techniques described in this chapter.

On the other hand, there are several ways to help yourself forget information. One is to choose to rely on an external memory aid, such as writing down a password or allowing your phone or internet browser to store the password for you; this decision tags the password as something that can be forgotten.

You can also choose to extinguish a memory. To snuff out a memory, every time it pops up in your mind, consciously and deliberately attempt to extinguish the memory as you would a candle flame. Slam on the mental brakes if the details of the memory start to come back into mind, and don't allow the reminiscence to continue. Picture the memory as a sandcastle being washed away by the waves, or a chalk drawing that you are erasing. Put some effort into this task, and use whatever metaphor seems appropriate.

BEWARE OF ILLUSIONS OF MASTERY

Have you ever studied hard and thought you knew the mate-rial only to find that, when faced with the test, meeting, or presentation, you couldn't remember the content you studied? Although there are a number of reasons this might occur, one of the most common is that you experienced the illusion that you mastered the material when you actually didn't.

One of the most common methods of studying is to highlight or underline your textbook, notes, or company prospectus and then to study for your test, meeting, or presentation by re-reading them. Unfortunately, this is one of the worst ways to study. Although it's important to identify the key passages in your reading—and it's good to highlight or underline those passages—*re-reading* the same material doesn't help it to get into your brain. It's not active enough. It doesn't take enough effort. And, not only does the material not get into your brain, because it's easier to re-read a chapter or prospectus than to read it for the first time, you have the *illusion* that you know the material when you actually don't.

So, if re-reading is not the right approach to studying, what is?

TEST YOURSELF

The best way to study is to test yourself. The act of retrieving a memory makes it easier to retrieve it again later. Look at your highlighted textbook, underlined notes, or marked-up prospectus. Turn each concept, idea, formula, pathway, vocabulary word, financial figure, or other information you need to learn into a flashcard with the question on one side and the answer on the other. Then test yourself with the flashcards. (Note that there are smartphone apps that have similar functions. As long as you can do the different types of testing and sorting that we describe, they should probably work as well as physical cards.)

As you are testing yourself, sort the cards into two piles, those in which you easily knew the answer, and those in which you didn't know the answer, got it wrong, struggled with it, or guessed. Test yourself again on the cards you had trouble with. Keep repeating the process, periodically re-studying the cards you knew well so you'll strengthen that knowledge too. Don't be afraid of making errors; as long as you check your answers and correct your mistakes, you will remember the correct information.

What if you're going to be taking an essay test? After you've mastered the material that will go into the essays with your flashcards, test yourself by writing practice essays. Your professor uses short-answer tests? Create some of those and practice. You're going to be presenting a slide deck in a meeting and you need to prepare for unanticipated questions? Enlist as many colleagues as you can to give you any and all possible questions that could come up, and study those as well.

Depending upon the material, you may also benefit by taking practice tests that others have developed. You might find relevant tests online or in books that will help test your knowledge and—particularly if explanations are provided—help you learn the material. One of the reasons that many people benefit from taking a class to improve their performance on the standardized tests that are used for entrance to colleges, graduate schools, and professional schools is that such classes typically emphasize testing, testing, and more testing.

SPACE OUT YOUR STUDYING— AVOID CRAMMING

In addition to testing yourself, it is critical to space out your studying over a number of sessions. How much should you space it out? Enough so that a little bit of forgetting occurs between sessions. Then the relearning takes more effort—which is the point. You may start spacing your studying by just a few minutes or an hour or two, but the interval should lengthen as you gain a better grasp on the material. Sleep is important, so spacing it out a day with sleep in between is generally good once you can remember the material for several hours. But don't stop there—revisit the material a week later, and once a month after that if you want to remember it for the year-end test (and for the rest of your life).

Lastly, avoid cramming (doing all your studying in a short period of time). Sometimes you can get away with cramming at the last minute, but more often you'll do poorly on the exam or in the meeting. Most importantly, the knowledge you learn by cramming will likely vanish completely in a few weeks. It is a poor way to study.

VARY YOUR STUDYING

To build not only a strong but also a detailed memory of whatever content you're trying to remember, it is important to study in multiple ways from multiple vantage points. For example, once you can generate all the answers to the questions on your flashcards, turn the cards around and see if you can generate all the questions from the answers. Think about the company from the perspective of the leadership, managers, frontline employees, customers, and stockholders. Imagine historical events from each group's point of view, not just those provided in the textbook, and think about any current-day parallels. When learning a biochemical pathway, think about different ways the system could break down and what consequences would arise.

INTERLEAVE YOUR STUDYING

Along with varying your learning by studying in multiple ways, it's beneficial to interleave these different types of studying. So, even better than first testing yourself on all the questions and then testing yourself on all the answers, take your flashcards and divide them into two piles. Turn one pile upside down (so that the questions are facing up on one pile and the answers are facing up on the other) and shuffle the cards back together. Now test yourself on all of the flashcards. Once you've done that, turn the cards over and do it again. In this way you're interleaving different types of problems that you're giving yourself to learn the material. Use these same principles for learning that doesn't lend itself to flashcards. It's better to work on problem types ABCDABCDABCD rather than AAABBBCCCDDD. So, to consolidate your understanding, solve one type of math problem and then another, rather than solving a set of problems that all require the same underlying concept or procedural technique.

STUDY UNDER DIFFERENT CONDITIONS

In order to be easily able to retrieve the material you're studying under any conditions, it's important to vary the conditions in which you're studying. For example, if you are studying advanced cardiac life support, it's important that you can quickly recall that material whenever you need it. So, study the material in the morning, afternoon, evening, and night. Study in your bedroom, the clinic, and the hospital. Quiz yourself on the material indoors and outside. The more you vary when and where you study, the more easily the material will come to mind in any context.

SOLVE THE PROBLEM FIRST, THEN LEARN HOW TO DO IT

Your teacher has assigned a series of problems you have to solve for your homework. The only issue is, you haven't yet learned how to solve these types of problems. Did your teacher make a mistake? Are they just being mean? Not at all. As counterintuitive as it may feel, you're more likely to remember material if you try to figure out how to solve the problem first—and then read the chapter telling you how to do it—than if you read the chapter first. Similarly, in the working world, it's best to first try solving most problems on your own, and then—after struggling with it for a bit—go to a colleague or your boss for help.

Of course, there has to be the possibility that you can solve the problem (or get close to the solution). The term we use for this type of "right-size" problem is *desirable difficulty*, meaning that it is possible to solve the problem with your existing knowledge and a lot of effort, so it's not too hard nor too easy. By trying to solve the problems from the homework or the project first, and then going back and reading the chapter or speaking with a colleague (and correcting your answers, as needed), you'll be putting in the effort you need to build a strong memory of the material.

STRATEGIES WHEN RETRIEVING MEMORIES

Stay Calm: Relax

You are already running late for your appointment when you realize you can't find your keys. Although it's natural to begin to panic, work to stay calm and relax. Stress will only make it more difficult for you to remember where you left your keys or to recall whatever material you're trying to bring to mind. Remember that retrieval failures are common and there's no need to get upset about them. Of course, it's easy to say you should stay calm, but harder to do in practice. We recommend a few basic approaches:

- Take one or two slow, deep breaths as you feel your belly expand. These large, slow breaths will trigger your parasympathetic nervous system, which will help you relax.
- Keep in mind that everyone has these retrieval failures, your difficulty is likely temporary, and the information you are seeking is likely to come to mind soon.
- Know that you have all the techniques we're about to describe at your fingertips to help you remember.

Once you are calm, you can begin to use the retrieval strategies outlined in this chapter.

Minimize Interference and Blocking

When you are struggling to retrieve information to answer a question, try to resist the natural urge to run through all possible specific answers—and never keep saying the wrong answer if you know it's wrong. Although well intentioned, these attempts will actually interfere with your retrieval and block the correct answer. So, if your friend asks you, "What's the name of that movie you were telling me about last week?" it won't generally help to go through your favorite movies of all time or the current movies playing (unless you already know it's likely to be on one of those lists). Running through those lists will just block the right answer.

Create General and Diverse Retrieval Cues

When searching for information from your memory that doesn't come easily, try bringing to mind broad and varied retrieval cues. Think of other things that you do know related to the information you're searching for. Or think of a time when you were discussing or learning the information. For example, if you're trying to recall which movie you were discussing with your friend, rather than run through a list of movies, try recalling other details and topics of the conversation you had that day. Think about the emotions you were experiencing and the expressions on your friend's face. These general and diverse cues will help you to recall the information you're looking for without blocking it.

Return to the Internal and External Context of Your Learning

Another good technique to recall information is to imagine yourself back in the same time and location you were in when you were learning the information in the first place. If you're looking for your keys, mentally retrace your steps when you got home. Also think about your internal context—how you were feeling—at the time. In doing so, you may then recall you were so thirsty that, keys in hand, you went right to the refrigerator to get a bottle of water. (Sure enough, there are your keys, sitting on the refrigerator shelf.) If you're having trouble recalling which colleague has the dairy allergy, think about where you were when you were having that conversation and other topics you discussed at the time.

If you're trying to bring material you've learned to mind when you're in the middle of an exam or presentation, mentally time travel and try to picture yourself back in your classroom, office, bedroom, or wherever you were when you were learning the material you're trying to retrieve. Visualize the textbook, homework assignments, prospectus, or websites you reviewed. If you studied to music, think of the tunes that you were listening to at the time. If you like to drink hazelnut coffee while studying, imagine that flavor in your mouth.

Protect Against False Memories

False memories are common. Remember that when you retrieve a memory you are actually reconstructing it. For this reason, it's easy for mistakes to become incorporated in your memory, such as two memories becoming mixed up with each other.

Evaluate the Details

The best way to avoid false memories is to evaluate the memory you have just retrieved. Is your memory vivid and full of sensory details? Although not a guarantee of authenticity, the more specific details that your memory contains, the more likely it is to be real and accurate. Memories (or parts of memories) that are vague and contain only general information may be false or distorted half-truths. For example, if you are asked if you went on Disney's Big Thunder Mountain Railroad ride, and you remember the loud cracking and clicking sounds that periodically occurred, and how parts of it vibrated and shook so much you thought it was going to shake apart your spine, these specific sensory details clue you that it's probably a real memory. But is it a memory of Thunder Mountain? It can be worth spending time searching for additional specific details to make sure that there wasn't another, similar rollercoaster, that was the source of your vivid memory. On the other hand, when asked about whether you went on the Haunted Mansion ride, if you think you did but can only remember it being a spooky ride in the dark, these vague and general notions suggest that it's as likely to be a false memory as a true one.

Could It Have Happened That Way?

Another way to evaluate whether a memory might be false is to compare its contents with factual information. For example, you may recall that you took your daughter to Star Wars: Galaxy's Edge at Disney World when she was 10 years old, but when you realize that it wasn't built until she was 12, you know that must have been a false, distorted, or otherwise mixed-up memory.

How Well Should You Remember This Content?

Perhaps a childhood friend says to you, "Remember when we went ice skating on that pond in sixth grade?" Simply thinking about this question might trigger you to have a vague memory of skating on a frozen pond with your friend in sixth grade. But is it really true? If you went ice skating on ponds dozens of times growing up, it will be difficult for you to sort out whether the particular memory you're bringing up is true or false. However, as we mentioned earlier in this chapter, things that are distinctive are easier to remember. For this reason, if you only skated on a pond once or twice in your life, these experiences would be distinctive, and you would be more likely to vividly recall the memory of skating on the pond with your friend if it had actually happened. In this case, despite your vague memory, you can respond, "No, I don't think that was me skating with you on the pond in sixth grade, because I'm sure I would have remembered that."

Did You Use Extra Effort? That Will Help for Next Time

Were you able to retrieve the memory you were looking for, but only with much effort and perhaps some of the techniques we outlined in this chapter? If so, that's great! The extra effort that you put in to recall that memory will help you retrieve it more easily next time.

WHAT ABOUT YOUR LEARNING STYLE?

Do you need to know your learning style to know the best way to study? No. Don't try to learn things by auditory or visual means alone. Everyone learns better when they draw on all their aptitudes. Although you may have a preference for how you like to learn new material, that doesn't mean that translates into how you are best able to learn. Be careful not to confuse learning that seems easy with learning that will stick with you. Don't forget that we remember things better when we put *effort* into them, not when they come easily.

What is important is that your learning matches the nature of what is being taught. For example, art history, anatomy, and geometry should be learned visually; literature, poetry, and music theory should be learned auditorily. For material that could be learned either way, although using both methods is always preferable, most studies show that, if you had to choose, learning visually produces the best retention of the material. For example, if you can turn spreadsheets into bar graphs, line graphs, pie charts, Pareto charts, and other visual displays, they will be easier to remember.

STUDY TOGETHER—AND ALONE

There are many benefits to studying in small groups. Critical thinking skills often increase as you learn from others how to get past sticking points and problem areas you may have faced alone. You may also better appreciate the breadth and depth of the material. Be careful, however, of studying for exams or preparing for presentations in a group if you alone will be required to recall all the information. Otherwise, in the middle of the exam or presentation, you may end up with the realization that although the group as a whole might have known the answer to the question, you as an individual do not. We therefore recommend that you study both in groups and by yourself—this way you get the best of both approaches.

SLEEP AS A STRATEGY

Whatever you are studying, you'll remember it better if you sleep after you put in effort to learn the material. So, if you have 10 hours of material to learn and 10 days to learn it, you'll master the material better and remember it longer if—in addition to everything we mentioned earlier in this chapter—you study the material an hour each day rather than cramming 10 hours the day prior to the exam. (Note that if the 10 hours of material are 10 unrelated units that don't build on each other, make sure you review some of the material you previously learned each day.)

It's also helpful to review the material shortly before bed—that will increase the chances that sleep will strengthen your memory for the material. If you enjoy listening to calm, relaxing music while you are studying, try listening to the same music while you are getting ready for sleep; this may also increase the chances that sleep will strengthen your memory for the material.

Don't stay up all night studying; you'll remember the information better if you give yourself time to sleep. And make sure you get enough sleep each night—the studies show that students who sleep well for several weeks prior to the exam do the best on it. Make sure you get enough sleep each night.

REFLECT UPON YOUR RETRIEVAL

Lastly, if you're trying to improve your memory abilities, it's worthwhile to reflect upon whether your memory worked for you at your recent client meeting, job interview, social event, or exam. Were you easily able to recall the names, dates, locations, and other material you wanted to? Or did you struggle—or fail—to retrieve the content you needed at the time? If you did well, congratulations! If not, using the list at the end of this chapter of all the different strategies we presented, write down whether you used each one a lot, a little bit, or not at all. Think about whether strategies you didn't use (or only used a little) might have enabled you to master the material better. Use that information for the next time you need to prepare for a meeting, presentation, exam, or interview.

What's that you're saying? You've been using all the strategies in this chapter but you're still struggling to remember names or the material you need to learn for your job or course? The information in Chapters 24 and 25 may be just what you're looking for.

USE STRATEGIES TO ENHANCE YOUR MEMORY ABILITIES

Now that you understand how your memory works and the different strategies available to you, pick the strategies that will best help you remember whatever material or experience you wish.

- Strategies when acquiring memories
  - Be motivated.
  - Align your in-the-moment goals with your memory goals.
  - Relax! Don't be anxious.
  - Use effort to do *FOUR* things.
    - **Focus** attention. Avoid distraction—don't multitask. Take breaks. Consider a cup of coffee (or tea). Use your senses. Create sensational mnemonics.
    - **Organize** and cluster. Chunk that information.
    - **Understand**. Build from the foundations up. Generate content.
    - **Relate**. Make associations. Create visual images.
  - Take ownership of your learning.
  - Make it distinctive: *Involve the senses. Use humor. Imbue it with emotion. Make it important to you.*
  - Acquire content in the way you will need to retrieve it.
  - Make acronyms.
- Choose whether you will remember or forget it.
- Beware of illusions of mastery.
- Test yourself.
- Space out your studying—avoid cramming.
- Vary your studying.
- Interleave your studying.
- Study under different conditions.
- Solve the problem first, then learn how to do it.
- Strategies when retrieving memories
  - Stay calm: Relax.
  - Minimize interference and blocking.
  - Create general and diverse retrieval cues.
  - Return to the internal and external context of your learning.
  - Protect against false memories: *Evaluate the details. Could it have happened that way? How well should you remember this content?*
  - Did you use extra effort? That will help for next time!

- Match your learning to the nature of what is being taught. *Learn visually and auditorily whenever possible.*
- Study together—and alone.
- Sleep as a strategy.
- Reflect upon your retrieval.

24

Remember names

You're chatting with some friends at a conference when a colleague
you've known for years walks up and enthusiastically says, "Hello,
so good to see you!" The conversation pauses and all eyes turn to
you expectantly while everyone waits for you to introduce her. You
open your mouth to respond—but you can't remember her name.

Has something like this happened to you? Or have you ever
introduced yourself to someone, they introduce themselves to
you in return, you begin talking, and—60 seconds later—you
realize you cannot remember their name?

Building on the basic strategies we've just reviewed in the last
chapter, we'll discuss how to solve both of these problems: how
to better learn new names and how to recall someone's name
that you know.

LEARN NAMES

Pay Attention

It sounds deceptively simple and obvious, but the first thing
you need to do in order to remember someone's name that you
are meeting is to pay attention to the name when they are saying it. Typically, you are paying attention to them—you're making eye contact, looking at the social cues in their face and body

language, closely examining their reactions to you, and thinking of what you are going to say next. With all this cognitive activity going on, it's no wonder that you forgot to pay attention to their *name*! So, when they say, "Hi, my name is Mary," stop the other cognitive activity going on in your head and pay attention to their name. (Are you having difficulty focusing your attention? Try improving your attention by practicing mindfulness as described in Chapter 21.) Once you've paid attention to their name, you need to firmly ensconce it in your memory.

Spell the Name

Whether it is a common name you've heard a hundred times or one you're hearing for the first time, try to spell the name. If you're not sure how to spell it, ask the person right then and there. For example, "It's nice to meet you, John . . . is that J-O-H-N or J-O-N for Jonathan?" "Great to meet you, Anahita . . . could you spell that for me? . . . Oh, I see, 'An-a-hi-ta,' thanks."

Repeat the Name

In addition to spelling the name, you want to repeat the name immediately after you've heard it. It's best to repeat the name aloud, such as saying, "Hi, Mary, it's nice to meet you. My name is Andrew." Or, if it wouldn't be appropriate to say the name aloud in that particular setting or point in the conversation, say the name silently to yourself.

You then want to repeat the name several times in the conversation. Sometimes you can say it aloud naturally: "I couldn't agree with you more, Mary." Otherwise, repeat the name silently to yourself as you think, "Mary made a great point there." Repeat the name again as you're saying goodbye: "It was nice to meet you, Mary." Then, as you're going to get a drink, think to yourself, "I just met Mary." As you are driving home that evening, run through the names of the people you met. Say to yourself, "I first met Mary, then Jon (J-O-N for Jonathan), and lastly Anahita (An-a-hi-ta)." And if you really want to remember their names for a long time, think about them again tomorrow, later that week, and perhaps a month or two after that.

Make a Remark About the Name

Another natural way to repeat the name is to say (or think) a remark about it. If you have a family member or friend with the same name, you can comment on that, such as, "One of my closest friends growing up was named Anahita."

Make an Association

Next, you want to make an association with the name. This association can be almost anything that will help you remember the name. If you have a family member or close friend with the same name, you can use that for the association. If the name naturally lends itself to an association, you can use that one (such as the first names Brooke, Daisy, and Rose, or the last names Baker, Cooper [barrel maker], and Smith [blacksmith]). We will often use famous people to make an association, such as Jonathan Swift for Jonathan and Muhammad Ali for Muhammad. If it is a name that you've never heard before or don't know its derivation, you can use the sounds of the name to make an association. For Anahita, perhaps you know it is the name of the Persian goddess of the waters and could use that imagery to remember the name; if you didn't know that association, you might think of *An A* (yes, the letter A) saying *hi* and then *ta*-ta. It doesn't matter if the association is logical, elegant, or wouldn't make sense to anyone but you.

Create an Image

Using your association, create a visual image. Remember that if the image is distinctive or silly, it will be even easier to remember. For Brooke, picture Brooke walking through a brook, getting their shoes all wet and muddy. You might want to imagine Daisy picking daisies—but to make it silly and distinctive, perhaps the daisies she is picking are growing out of her head. Perhaps Rose is picking roses and her fingers are all bandaged because of the thorns. For Baker, Cooper, and Smith, you can picture them working as a baker, barrel maker, and blacksmith. For Jonathan, because of your association with Jonathan Swift, you might picture Jonathan standing in tall grass that extends past his head (which happened to the protagonist in Swift's most famous book). For Muhammad, you might picture him wearing Ali's red boxing gloves—which clash wonderfully with the suit and tie Muhammad is actually wearing. For Anahita, as mentioned in the last section, you might picture as *An A* (a gigantic letter A) waving *hi* with one hand and *ta*-ta with the other hand (yes, this letter has hands).

Find the Facial Feature

Next you want to find a prominent facial feature, an aspect of their face that you can notice the next time you see them. Don't focus on features that are likely to change each time you see them, such as their hairstyle or glasses or makeup, but on more permanent characteristics. Perhaps they have freckles, a mole, or something distinctive about their nose, ears, or eyebrows. Perhaps their face shape brings to mind an association, just as in *The Wizard of Oz*, people's characteristics conjured a lion, a tin man, and a scarecrow.

Connect Your Image to the Facial Feature

Now you want to connect the image you created to the facial feature you selected. Does Brooke's face remind you of a lion? Think of them as a lion walking through the brook. Does Jonathan have a cleft in his chin? Picture the grass growing up past his face and creating that cleft. Are Daisy's ears distinctive? Picture tiny daisies growing out of her ears, and she's plucking those. What about Anahita? Because our mnemonic for her name uses a gigantic letter A, consider finding an A on her face, such as the A-shaped triangle formed by her nose, and picture her nose as *an A* waving *hi* and *ta*-ta. Have fun making these connections and remember that if it is distinctive and silly it will be easier to remember.

Depending on the context in which you're meeting people, it can be a fun icebreaker to work collaboratively to create these types of mental images. For instance, Elizabeth's students and colleagues often want to remember her last name, Kensinger, and not to confuse it with similar last names, such as Kensington or Kissinger. Elizabeth happens to have a set of moles on her face and neck that follow a similar pattern to the Big Dipper constellation (at least, similar enough to be useful in these types of mnemonics). After pointing those out, she'll let people's imaginations get to work. One of her favorites is a student who made the Ken-singer association especially strong by imagining a miniaturized Elizabeth singing a duet with a Ken doll, standing on a star-shaped stage against a backdrop of a starry night.

Add Other Connections

Once you've solidified the connection between the individual's name and their face using the image you created, you can connect other pieces of information as well. Want to remember that Daisy is an attorney? Picture the daisies coming out of her ears having yellow gavels in their centers. To recall that Jonathan has three children, picture them climbing up the large blades of grass that surround him. To remember that Muhammad is a professor at Harvard, picture him, in his suit with Ali's boxing gloves on, sitting in place of the statue of John Harvard in Harvard Yard.

Repeat the Connection

Remember we mentioned earlier that you want to repeat their name several times in the conversation and afterwards, either aloud or to yourself? You also want to picture the image you created and its connection to their face each time you repeat the name. Repeatedly connecting the image with their face will help you to build a strong memory.

Effort Is Good and Practice Makes Perfect

Does all this seem like a lot of work just to remember a name? That's good! The more effort you put into creating a memory, the more likely you will be able to retrieve it when you need it. In addition, the more you try to use this and other strategies to aid your memory, the more these strategies will become automatic. Soon you'll find that you've gotten into the habit of repeating names, making associations, creating images, and connecting the image to facial features.

RETRIEVE NAMES

If you've learned someone's name well using the techniques we've just described, we suspect it will be relatively easy for you to retrieve their name. But if you run into one of the several thousand people you met before you read this book, you may need some strategies to help you retrieve their name. Here they are.

Relax

Remember, there are few things as detrimental to memory retrieval as feeling stress. So, it's important to relax and not get nervous about the fact that you're struggling to recall their name and about to experience an embarrassing situation. Use the approaches to calm yourself outlined in Chapter 23. If the name is still not coming to mind, just focus on being friendly and relaxed. The name may come to you automatically once you're relaxed.

Minimize Interference and Blocking

If a wrong name comes to mind that you believe is close to the right one, resist the urge to continue saying it to yourself—that will only block the correct name and interfere with its retrieval. So, after saying, "Is it Molly? No, that's not right. What about Marie? No, that's not right either," don't keep saying, "OK, so it's not Molly or Marie . . . not Molly or Marie . . . what could it be if it's not Molly or Marie?"

Generate General Retrieval Cues

Instead of repeating the wrong name, think about the other things you know about the person. Perhaps you can recall some of what you spoke about when you last met. Think about where they work, where they live, what hobbies they have, which sports teams they like, or their children. Think about who introduced you to them. Any of these more general retrieval cues may activate the semantic network that triggers the retrieval of their name.

Think of When You Were with Them

Time-travel in your mind to where you were and what you were doing when you first met them, or when you last saw them and used their name. Picture the location, context, ambiance, music, and other people present. Try to match your mood and thoughts at the time as well. For example, recalling that you last spoke to them excitedly when your favorite sports team was in the playoffs may help the name spring to mind.

Use the Alphabet

One way to generate a helpful retrieval cue that is not dependent on your memory of the person is to run through the alphabet. Oftentimes the first letter of their name is a sufficient cue to allow you to retrieve the rest of it. Going through the alphabet is also one good way to stop yourself from blocking the name if those intrusive wrong names keep coming to mind.

Review Names Ahead of Time

If you are going to be attending an event where there will be a bunch of people whose names you "should" know but may not have on the tip of your tongue, it's often a good idea to review their names (and perhaps other information) ahead of time. For example, if you are attending one of your partner's work parties, you may see people you've known for a long time but haven't seen for a year or more (and never knew very well). To facilitate your recall during the party, you might want to spend a few minutes with your partner earlier that evening talking about which of their colleagues you're likely to see at the party as well as a couple pieces of information about each one, such as where they live and how old their children are.

If you're going to a reunion, you can review yearbook photos of your old friends. It's then particularly helpful to group them by how you might have known them: math club, marching band, soccer team, history class, and so forth. You can also use social media to make sure you know how they look now. Lastly, you can use any—or all—of the memory techniques we describe in Chapter 23 to help you learn a list of names before an event.

Still Can't Recall Their Name? Just Ask Them

Lastly, there is nothing so terrible about not being able to remember someone's name, even if you should know it. As we mentioned, retrieval failures happen to everyone. Just ask them for their name. And—now that they've told you—use the techniques in this chapter to solidify it in your brain so you'll remember it next time.

YOU CAN IMPROVE YOUR MEMORY FOR NAMES

Although few of us learn and retrieve names automatically and effortlessly, it isn't that difficult to improve these abilities. It simply takes some direct effort.

- To learn names
  - Pay attention.
  - Spell the name.
  - Repeat the name.
  - Make a remark about the name.
  - Make an association.
  - Create an image.
  - Find the facial feature.
  - Connect your image to the facial feature.
  - Add other connections.
  - Repeat the connection.
  - Effort is good and practice makes perfect.
- To retrieve names
  - Relax.
  - Minimize interference and blocking: *Don't keep saying the wrong name!*
  - Generate general retrieval cues.
  - Think of when you were with them.
  - Use the alphabet.
  - Review names ahead of time.
  - Still can't recall their name? Just ask them!

25

Advanced strategies and mnemonics

In her second career, your friend is studying to become a massage therapist. She shares with you that she's in a panic because she's concerned that she'll never be able to remember the names and actions of all muscles she needs to memorize for her degree. You say some encouraging words but silently wonder how anyone could remember all those muscles—especially after age 40! You run into her again a few months later and ask her how the studying is going. She laughs and tells you that she memorized all those muscles ages ago using a memory strategy.

Do you need to remember the 200+ bones and 600+ muscles in the human body? Perhaps you would you like to remember each of your 16-digit credit card numbers in your head—plus the expiration date and three-digit security code. How about the prime numbers from one to 100? What about all of your passwords for various websites, computer programs, and phone apps? Maybe you'd just like to remember your holiday shopping list without writing it down. In this chapter we'll teach you how to remember all these things plus directions, speeches, playing cards, and more.

A couple of notes. First, these strategies build on those presented in Chapters 23 and 24, so please read those chapters first

343

if you haven't already. Second, we don't call these strategies "advanced" for nothing: Several of them require you to learn whole new organizational frameworks, systems, and schemas. That's right—in order to memorize what you want to remember, you have to first memorize whole new systems of remembering. We understand that not everyone is interested in doing that, which is why we put these advanced strategies at the end. Feel free to skim them or skip them altogether if you wish.

METHOD OF LOCI OR MEMORY PALACE

Let's begin with one of the oldest and best techniques, the *method of loci*, also called a *memory palace*, developed by the ancient Greeks more than 2,500 years ago. As you will see, this technique uses many of those we have discussed, including building on existing knowledge, making associations, and using visualization, distinctiveness, emotion, and humor. The basic idea is simple: Picture a structure or other location that you know extremely well, such as your home. Think about how you might walk through your home so that you would visit each room once (it's OK if you need to backtrack down a hallway). Don't forget basements, bathrooms, hall closets, attics, and so forth. Once you have your structure and route—which should always be the same—you mentally put the things that you would like to remember into the rooms of your house, arranged in the order that you would like to retrieve them.

For example, perhaps you want to memorize your grocery list. Easy. Just open your front door and start your journey inside your memory palace. Imagine an apple in your foyer. But we need to make that apple memorable, so picture yourself stepping on the apple, it rolling out from under your feet, and you almost fall. (Whew, that was close!) Then you turn left into the living room, where you find a bowl of chocolate pudding and—oh no—someone left chocolate pudding handprints all over the white sofa! Then you turn right into your dining room.

There, in the center of the table, is a beautiful roast chicken. But wait—as you bend over to inspect it, you can hear that it's clucking. Well, this is a bit macabre, but it seems to be clucking happily, and now it's memorable. You make your way into the kitchen and—to your surprise—find yourself ankle deep in mud. Your kitchen floor has been transformed into a garden with beautiful tomatoes growing on a vine. OK, you need to get yourself cleaned up, and so you make your way to the bathroom where you can wash off the mud. Although there might be better detergents for this purpose, all you can find is hand soap; in fact, the entire tub is filled with hand soap—just what you need from the market. You dip your hand in and clean yourself up before moving down the hall to your bedroom. You put your hand on your bedroom doorknob and notice, as you're turning the knob, that it feels cold, like ice. You enter your bedroom and find it has been transformed into a walk-in freezer with little green balls everywhere. A closer look reveals the little balls to be frozen peas. So, we've finished the tour of our little memory palace and now we can remember to purchase the following items: an apple, chocolate pudding, a roast chicken, tomatoes, hand soap, and frozen peas.

Specific Quantities

What's that you say? How will you remember you need a dozen apples? Perhaps, when you walk in the foyer, the dozen apples are in a large egg carton—but when you approach them they launch themselves out of the carton and onto the floor (where you step on them, like before, and almost fall).

Enlarge Your Palace

What now? You have 24 more items to get at the market and you don't have any more rooms in your house? Not a problem.

In addition to the sofa (with chocolate pudding handprints), your living room has an armchair, a rocking chair, a rug, a coffee table, a liquor cabinet, an end table, and a picture on the wall. You can put the lemons and limes on the armchair (someone cut them in half and squeezed them, staining the chair yellow and green), the eggs are in the rocking chair (rocking back and forth, causing the eggs to slide off and crack on the floor), there's a jar of salsa on the rug (on its side, lid off, salsa spilling onto the rug), there are mounds of coffee grains covering the coffee table, a six-pack of beer is on the liquor cabinet (arranged in a pyramid: three on the bottom, two in the middle, one on top), your end table looks white because it is wrapped in toilet paper like a furniture mummy, and there's a bottle of glass cleaner with its handle hanging onto the top of the framed picture—next to a large area of the picture that has been erased with the cleaner.

Now we're up to a total of 14 items and we haven't even included the different areas of your dining room, kitchen, or bathroom, nor the closet and furniture of your bedroom. It should be no problem to get to at least 52 specific locations in your memory palace. (Why 52? So you can put a playing card in each location—something you'll need to do if you want to enter the USA Memory Championship, like Joshua Foer did in his book, *Moonwalking with Einstein*.)[1]

MARK TWAIN'S MEMORY

Samuel Clemens, better known as Mark Twain, had a notoriously poor memory. One of his biographers wrote that he became lost in his own neighborhood and failed to recognize pictures that had been hanging in his house for years. Perhaps because of his poor memory, he spent time learning—and then developing and publishing—various systems for remembering history, his lectures, and other information.[2]

In one of his first successes, he taught his children to remember the English monarchs using 817 feet of his driveway. At the start he hammered in a peg and labeled it *1066: William the*

Conqueror. Each monarch after William had another peg measured out (1 foot per year), hammered in, and labeled, with the final peg being 1883 (the current year). His children had great fun racing from peg to peg and shouting out the monarchs' names and years they ascended the throne. Although this game was a successful mnemonic technique for his children, Twain's memory-enhancing publications were not—none made a profit.

Twain was successful, however, in his use of little pictures to remember the nightly lectures he gave when going on book tours. He would draw a haystack to remind him of Carson Valley, a rattlesnake to remind him of a strange and violent wind that blew from the Sierra Nevadas, and a lightning bolt to remind him of the weather in San Francisco. Each picture would be a cue for him to tell a particular story as part of his lecture. Because he had a fear of losing his lecture notes—which happened to him once—he then memorized the pictures and threw them away, so there was nothing to lose.[3]

Twain was able to remember the pictures and their order by linking them to his own version of a memory palace. He used the locations of items on a dinner table, such as napkin, fork, plate, knife, spoon, saltcellar, butter plate, and so on.[2] And so, with this method, the great storyteller was able to spin his yarns, without notes, night after night.

POWERPOINT PICTURES, LECTURES, AND SPEECHES

You can use Twain's system of little pictures to help you remember each point you would like to make in a slide presentation. Everyone knows you should not simply read whole sentences off slides. Most people turn their points into brief bulleted phrases that cue them to talk about those points. Instead of words or phrases, try using a relevant picture to cue you to talk about each point. Not only will you remember them better, but your audience will remember your points better, too. To give a lecture or a speech without slides, simply put each picture into your memory palace or chain them together in order as described in the next section. Voilà! You've got your speech memorized.

CHAINING

Remembering topics and other items by pictures generally works extremely well. To make sure that you don't forget any of the pictures (and thus the items they represent), memorizing them in an order is key. One good method to do so is to use your memory palace, as we described earlier. Sometimes, however, it's simpler and easier to use *chaining*. In chaining, you simply connect one picture to the next in some visual, distinctive, and often humorous way.

Let's say that you have a dozen items you need to pick up to prepare for a birthday party: bananas (you're making banana splits for dessert), a wristwatch (your present), a cake (from the bakery), birthday candles, some ribbon, a birthday card, balloons, your tablecloth (from the cleaners), champagne, plastic champagne glasses, purple napkins, and a large tent (in case it rains). There are a million ways to chain these together; here is one way off the top of our heads. You start with a *banana*, and the banana has a *wristwatch* around it. As you look at the dial, you can see the face of the watch is actually a miniature *cake*, and the hands are lit *birthday candles*. When the hands reach 12, they reach a *ribbon*—which catches on fire! The long ribbon burns until it reaches a *birthday card*, and that catches on fire, too. Luckily, a water *balloon* bursts on the card, putting the fire out, but now the *tablecloth* (that the card was on) is soaked. As you start to take the soaked tablecloth off the table, you forgot that there were open *champagne* bottles on it—they tip over and the champagne starts flowing onto the floor. In a flash, you grab your *plastic champagne glasses* and start to catch as much of the bubbly liquid as you can. Unfortunately, there's still a lot of it on the floor, and so you use your *purple napkins* to soak it up. One of the napkins absorbs more and more liquid and starts to swell and grow until soon it is the size of a *large tent*.

Now close your eyes: Can you list off the 12 items in order as the pictures follow one after another in your mind? Make up your own chain of connections for any list of items and the effort you put into the chain will help you to remember them. Note that you can do 100 items or more this way and—as long as each image is vivid and distinct—you'll be able to remember them all in order. This is one way that you can remember the 200+ bones and 600+ muscles in the human body. Make up a picture that goes with each name, such as a river delta for the *deltoid*, the rushing water making it hard to ride your bicycle (for *biceps*), so you jump off your bicycle and onto a triceratops (for *triceps*) who was going the other way (triceps and biceps have opposite actions), and so forth.

NUMBERS

There are a few different ways to remember numbers. In Chapter 23 we described chunking, explaining how you can take a 16-digit credit card number and break it down into shorter numbers that can represent dates, numbers on players' jerseys, or other numbers that might be meaningful to you and therefore easier to remember than 16 random digits. But now that you know how to remember images in order using either your memory palace or by chaining them together, you're ready to learn a more powerful tool.

Phonetic Number System
The phonetic number system was invented by the French mathematician and astronomer Pierre Hérigone in about 1570,

and further developed by others over the next 450 years.[4] The basic idea is simply to turn numbers into the sounds of specified consonants, and then you add vowels to turn the string of consonants into words. Next turn the words into images and memorize the images in order by chaining or using your memory palace.

Here are the numbers, their specific consonant sounds, and some suggestions as to how to remember which consonants go with which number:[5]

1 = t (or **d, th**): one downstroke (vertical stroke of your pen), or a horizontal 1 on a vertical 1

2 = n: two downstrokes

3 = m: three downstrokes, and an m on its side is a 3

4 = r: final sound of four, or capital R as a golfer about to drive, yelling "fore!"

5 = l: Roman numeral L is 50; hold up your left hand, fingers together, thumb outstretched, and you'll make an L with your five fingers

6 = j (or **sh, ch, soft g**): 6 and letter J are almost mirror images

7 = k (or **hard c, hard g, q, sometimes x**): you can form a K with two 7's

8 = f (or **v, ph**): script f has two loops like an 8

9 = p (or **b**): 9 and P are almost mirror images

0 = s (or **soft c, z, sometimes x**): think of the first sound in zero, cipher, xylophone*

Note that the reason some numbers, such as 1, can be represented by either t or d is that these sounds are very similar, using the same mouth position, and differing only whether the sound is voiced or not. These pairings of letters are logical and not arbitrary. Vowels (a, e, i, o, u) and letters w, h, y have no number value. Silent letters have no value because they make

---

*. From *Ageless Memory* by Harry Lorayne, copyright © 2008. Reprinted by permission of Black Dog & Leventhal, an imprint of Hachette Book Group, Inc.

no sound (knee = 2, whereas kin = 72). Double letters that make one sound have one value.

Passcodes and Credit Card Numbers

Let's start with some short numbers to warm up before we tackle longer ones. Suppose you were staying in a rental apartment that had a four-digit code that needed to be pressed on a keypad to unlock the door: 2921. Using the phonetic number system, 2/9/2/1 becomes n/p or b/n/t, d, or th. Take those letters and see if you can make one or more words by inserting vowels in between them. One possibility would be "knob knot" and the picture of the door*knob* made up of a *knot* to help remember the door code. But you could use "nip need," "knob kneed," or "no beneath" if you wished, because all of those two-word phrases would represent the numbers 2921. (Don't forget that silent letters have no points, which is why knob = 29, dumb = 13, and crack = 747.)

Now that you understand the principle, let's tackle the same 16-digit credit card number we used in Chapter 23. You first turn the numbers 1350246791181012 into letters:

t,d,th/m/l/s,c,z,x/n/r/j,sh,ch,g/k,c,g,q,x/p,b/t,d,th/t,d,th/f,v,ph/
t,d,th/s,c,z,x/t,d,th/n

Then you turn the letters into words. Don't forget that it is the sounds, not the actual letters, that count. Here are the words that we came up with after working on it for a few minutes:

Thumb loosener Jack putted foods tin.

Finally, you turn the words into images. If the images are all nouns, you can use chaining (our favorite for this purpose) or your memory palace. In this case we happened upon a silly sentence that lends itself to imagery. We picture a golfer, nicknamed "*thumb loosener Jack*" because he sticks his thumb in the air and wiggles it around as he loosens it up, having just *putted* various *foods* in the *tin* cup, which is now filled with eggs, oranges, and onions.

50 Digits of Pi

Ready for a challenge? Let's memorize the first 50 digits of pi:

3.14159265358979323846264338327950288419716939937 51

Perhaps start by chunking it a bit to make it easier to handle:

3.141 5926 5358 9793 2384 6264 3383 2795 0288 4197 1693 9937 51

Now turn the numbers into letters, keeping in mind the rules explained earlier about hard and soft c's, g's, and x's:

m/t,d,th/r/t,d,th/ l/p,b/n/j,sh,ch,g/ l/m/l/f,v,ph/ p,b/k,c,g,q,x/ p,b/m/ n/m/f,v,ph/r/ j,sh,ch,g/n/j,sh,ch,g/r/ m/m/f,v,ph/m/ n/ k,c,g,q,x/p,b/l/   s,c,z,x/n/f,v,ph/f,v,ph/   r/t,d,th/p,b/k,c,g,q,x/ t,d,th/j,sh,ch,g/p,b/m/ p,b/p,b/m/k,c,g,q,x/ l/t,d,th

Next turn the letters into words, keeping in mind that you don't need to respect the four-letter groupings; that was just to make the numbers and letters easier to handle:

My torte lap nosh lamb loaf Puck poem gnome over chain chair mom foam neck balls enough for Top Cat shape map bomb killed

Coming up with these words took us around 25 minutes. Notice that "enough" = 28 because the "ough" makes an "f" sound.

Once you have your words, you need to either chain them together or put them in your memory palace. We chained the words into a silly image:

I'm pulling *my torte* into my *lap* to eat a little *nosh*. A *lamb* walks up (attracted by the food), so I give the lamb a *loaf* of bread. *Puck*, that mischievous fairy, eats the loaf while reciting a *poem*, which attracts a *gnome*, who falls *over* a *chain* and into a *chair* in which your *mom* was sitting. Your mom gets up from the chair, sprays *foam* on her *neck*, which falls off in little *balls enough for Top Cat* to *shape* them into a *map*—but then a *bomb* went off and *killed* the cat.

We confess it's not the most concise, coherent, or cat-friendly story—you might be able to do much better with the words or the images. But it actually works for us to remember all 50 digits of pi. You can use the same method to memorize the next 50, 100, or 1,000 digits if you wish. It's only limited by your imagination.

PEG METHOD FOR LISTS

Sometimes you want to remember items associated with a specific number. For example, you might need to remember that your daughter's shoe size is 7½, your history class starts at 2 p.m., and you need to take your asthma medication at 10 a.m. To memorize these, we recommend using the *peg method*. The peg method associates each number with a word. Most memory gurus will use words based on the phonetic number system, such as the Lorayne list below:[5]

Phonetic Number Peg List

0 = s, z = zoo
1 = t, d, th = tie
2 = n = Noah
3 = m = ma
4 = r = rye
5 = l = law
6 = j, sh, ch = shoe
7 = k, c, g = cow
8 = f, v = ivy
9 = p, b = bee
10 = t + s = toes
11 = tide
12 = tin
13 = tomb
14 = tire
15 = tail
16 = dish
17 = dog

18 = dove
19 = tub
20 = nose†

and so forth.

For *ma* you might imagine your mother or the painting of Whistler's mother. For *law* you might picture a gavel or blind justice holding scales. Although we stopped at 20, because you know the phonetic number system, you can easily create your own peg list up to 100 (or 1,000) if you wish.

If you're not into the phonetic number system, you might prefer an easier-to-remember list based on rhyming. Here is a rhyming peg list from the book *Make It Stick*:[6]

Rhyming Peg List

1 = bun
2 = shoe
3 = tree
4 = store
5 = hive
6 = tricks
7 = heaven
8 = gate
9 = twine
10 = pen
11 = penny-one, setting sun
12 = penny-two, airplane glue
13 = penny-three, bumble-bee

and so forth.

Once you know your pegs, you can just make a silly image to associate what you are trying to remember with the appropriate peg. So, to remember your history class starts at 2 p.m., using the phonetic peg you can picture *Noah*'s ark sailing into your

†. From *Ageless Memory* by Harry Lorayne, copyright © 2008. Reprinted by permission of Black Dog & Leventhal, an imprint of Hachette Book Group, Inc.

history classroom, and using the rhyming peg you can imagine your history classroom with *shoes* everywhere like a shoe store. To remember that you need to take your asthma medication at 10 a.m., picture that you're holding your inhaler with your *toes* (phonetic) or puncturing your inhaler with a *pen* (rhyming) to get the medicine out.

What about remembering that your daughter's shoe size is 7½? Or if your meeting is at 4:15 or 3:45 p.m.? For half, you can add the image of a half an apple, sliced down from top to bottom so the stem and the seeds are showing. For a quarter past the hour (or just ¼) add the image of a quarter (the coin), and for a quarter to the hour (or just ¾) add the image of a pizza with one large slice eaten so that it is three-quarters complete, just missing the upper left quadrant (missing from 9 to 12 if it was a clock). So, to remember that your daughter's shoe size is 7½, picture her riding a cow (phonetic 7), which is eating an apple half while standing in your daughter's favorite pair of shoes (which are now all muddy). Or, if you prefer the rhyming list, picture your daughter wearing sparkly, magical shoes that raise her up in the air and into heaven, while she is eating an apple half.

LETTERS

Perhaps you need to remember a series of letters that don't necessarily form words, such as stock market symbols. One way to do this is to make up an image for each letter of the alphabet, such as *apple* for *A*, *bee* for *B*, *cat* for *C*, *dog* for *D*, *elephant* for *E*, and so on. Then, by forming a silly image chained together, you can easily remember short or long strings of letters. This is also helpful for memorizing passwords.

PASSWORDS

Speaking of passwords, by combining the phonetic number system and images for each letter, you can memorize almost any combination of numbers and letters in your various passwords. Chain them together to form an image of your password and connect it the application or website it is for. You can even design your password so that it reminds you of the website. For example, what would you associate with the password 8a0e9o7? Using the phonetic number system, you could read this as FaSePoK or, even better, FaCeBoK or Facebook. Similar, 1wi11e4 would be TwiTTeR (note that all three t's are pronounced) and i201a74a3 would be iNSTa-GRaM. What's that you're saying? Now I've told everyone your passwords? So, give them unique, personal twists. Use 9o78a0e (bookface) for Facebook. Or ae1wi11e4 for Andrew and Elizabeth's Twitter account. Use 3o27eY as your password for your local zoo website (we'll let you figure this one out).

PLAYING CARDS

From bridge to poker to gin rummy, in most card games it is beneficial to remember which cards were played. But there are 52 of them—that's a lot to remember. How to remember them? By using images, of course. In the following table is a list of images from Harry Lorayne (with a few modifications from us)[‡] based on the phonetic number system.[5] The idea is simple. For ace through 10, the first consonant is the first consonant of the suit: c for clubs, h for hearts, s for spades, and d for diamonds. The second consonant sound uses the phonetic number system, so for *ace* (which is really *1*) you add *t*, *d*, or *th*. For *2* you add *n*. For *3* you add *m*, and so on.

The jacks are just images of suit itself (club, heart, spade, diamond), but make them actual pictures, not the stylized

‡. From *Ageless Memory* by Harry Lorayne, copyright © 2008. Reprinted by permission of Black Dog & Leventhal, an imprint of Hachette Book Group, Inc.

symbols. So, picture an anatomical heart for jack of hearts, imagine a spade you'd use as a shovel for jack of spades, and so forth. For the queens, we let the iconic queen of hearts be simply "queen" and have the others begin with their suit letter and rhyme with queen. For the kings, we again have them begin with their suit letter and have them end *ng* or *nk*, remembering that a *k* and hard *g* are phonetically similar.

	Clubs	Hearts	Spades	Diamonds
Ace	Cat	Hat	Suit	Date
2	Can	Hen	Sun	Dune
3	Comb	Ham	Sum	Dam
4	Core	Hare	Sore	Door
5	Coal	Hail	Sail	Doll
6	Cash	Hash	Sash	Dash
7	Cog	Hog	Sock	Dock
8	Cuff	Hoof	Safe	Dive
9	Cup	Hub	Soap	Deb
10	Case	Hose	Sews	Dice
Jack	Club	Heart	Spade	Diamond
Queen	Cream	Queen	Steam	Dream
King	King	Hang	Sing	Drink

Once you have the images memorized, you can put the cards on your pegs as they are being played in each suit, allowing you to both count the cards in each suit as well as know which ones went by. You can also mutilate each card as it goes by, so you know which have been discarded and, by process of elimination, which ones are left. For the next hand, burn each card image in fire. The drown each in water. Then knife each card into little pieces. Then puncture each card. Then put a fork through each card. And so forth.

We know this all sounds like a lot of work, but you can start small and build up. Begin by just memorizing the aces one week, then kings the next, queens after that, and so forth. In 3 months, you'll have them memorized.

DIRECTIONS

Do you really need to use mnemonics for directions? Can't you use phone apps for that? Well, there are plenty of rural regions in which the apps don't work and, in some cities, tall buildings can block GPS signals and give you incorrect locations. For these reasons, it's good to have a system to be able to remember directions. Here's one that works with the phonetic number system and peg list.

Assign images you'll remember for *right, left, north, south, east, west,* such as *elephant, donkey, north pole with stripes, penguin, chopsticks,* and *cowboy hat,* respectively. If someone says, "Make a left, drive 10 blocks, make a right, 2 more blocks, make another right, then 4 blocks, and it's on the left," you can form the following chain of images: A *donkey* is turning left, and you're riding it, steering it with your *toes* (10) for 10 blocks. You jump off, and see an *elephant* turning right with *Noah* (2) riding on it. You run alongside and watch Noah riding for 2 blocks, and then you see a second *elephant* (this one is a baby elephant) that is turning right. You put a bag of *rye* (4) grain on the baby elephant. You lead it 4 blocks, and then see a *donkey* up ahead on the left, standing at your destination.

Or perhaps you're driving from the Salt Lake City Airport to Park City, Utah. You need to take the I-15 S to I-80 E to Exit 145, and then continue on UT-244 S. You can picture a gigantic eye (I) with a *penguin* (south) coming out of the pupil, *tail* (15) first, and the penguin drives through the pupil of another *eye* (I), where it leaves as you come to a woman wearing a *fez* (80) eating with *chopsticks* (east). She gets in and you drive her until you see a *troll* (145) telling you to take this exit, as it brings you *nearer* (244) to *Utah* (UT).

LAST WORDS: DISTINCTIVE IMAGES ARE MEMORABLE

The ancient Latin book *Rhetorica ad Herennium* sums up this chapter well in regard to what type of images should be used as mnemonics:

Now nature herself teaches us what we should do. When we see in everyday life things that are petty, ordinary, and banal, we generally fail to remember them, because the mind is not being stirred by anything novel or marvelous. But if we see or hear something exceptionally base, dishonorable, extraordinary, great, unbelievable, or laughable, that we are likely to remember a long time. Accordingly, things immediate to our eye or ear we commonly forget; incidents of our childhood we often remember best. Nor could this be so for any other reason than that ordinary things easily slip from the memory while the striking and novel stay longer in mind.[7]

This quotation reminds us that the images you create as mnemonics should be exceptional and distinctive in some way, as their distinctiveness makes them memorable.

After reading this book, you now understand a great deal about *why* distinctive images are memorable. You know that such images allow your hippocampus to build strong memories that are then tagged for prioritization, so the memories will be easier to reassemble in the future.

Whether you read this book for a school assignment, because you wanted to improve your memory, or just for enjoyment, we hope that it met your expectations. We also hope that—even if you don't recall all the specific details—you will remember the gist of the information we presented.

USE ADVANCED STRATEGIES AND MNEMONICS

You now have the full array of memory aids, strategies, and mnemonics available to you so that you are armed with the tools to memorize just about anything you would like to. Consider these advanced tools any time you need to memorize tens or hundreds of items.

- Use the method of loci, your memory palace.
- Use pictures to cue you.
- Chain images together.
- For lectures and speeches, chain images or use your memory palace.
- Use the phonetic number system:
  ○ 1 = t, d, th; 2 = n; 3 = m; 4 = r; 5 = l; 6 = j, sh, ch, soft g; 7 = k, hard c, hard g, q, hard x; 8 = f, v, ph; 9 = p, b; 0 = s, soft c, z, soft x.
- Use peg lists:
  ○ Phonetic number peg list: 0 = zoo, 1 = tie, 2 = Noah, 3 = ma, 4 = rye, 5 = law, 6 = shoe, 7 = cow, 8 = ivy, 9 = bee, 10 = toes, 11 = tide, 12 = tin, 13 = tomb, 14 = tire, 15 = tail, 16 = dish, 17 = dog, 18 = dove, 19 = tub, 20 = nose, and so on.
  ○ Rhyming peg list: 1 = bun; 2 = shoe; 3 = tree; 4 = store; 5 = hive; 6 = tricks; 7 = heaven; 8 = gate; 9 = twine; 10 = pen; 11 = penny-one, setting sun; 12 = penny two, airplane glue; 13 = penny-tree, bumble-bee; and so on.
- Use images for letters:
  ○ A = apple, B = bee, C = cat, D = dog, E = elephant, and so on.
- Remember passwords by combining the phonetic number system and images for letters.
- Use images for playing cards based on the phonetic number system.
- For directions, use images, the phonetic number system, and chaining.
- Remember: distinctive images are memorable.

Afterword

Before we end our journey together, we have two requests to make of you.

First, if you haven't done so while reading the book, take a moment to jot down a few important takeaways that you would like to remember from the content we've presented. Use some of the strategies we've described to commit those takeaways to memory. Consult your notes again tomorrow, next week, and next month, so that you will be able to take these lessons with you for the rest of your life.

Second, if you were unsatisfied with your memory in some way when you picked up this book, take a moment to write down at least one tangible method of how you will now approach a memory-related task using a new and better technique. Perhaps you are a student who will map out your semester in a way that carves out spaced study time. Possibly you are beginning a new job and will adopt some of the strategies outlined to learn the names of your new coworkers. Maybe you are a parent who will download a new to-do list or calendar application so that you can reserve your mental resources for those memory tasks that are not so easy to offload. Possibly you are a retiree who will prioritize setting aside 30 minutes a day for exercise or to resume a hobby you used to enjoy.

We ask you to do these things so that the information contained in this book will be freed from its covers and launched into your daily life. We hope that—even as today fades into yesterday—the takeaways you've learned and the goals you've set will become built into your memory structures and not be forgotten.

Tips to remember better

USE MEMORY AIDS

- Five general principles:
  - Be organized.
  - Be ready.
  - Don't delay.
  - Keep it simple.
  - Develop routines.
- A place for everything and everything in its place.
- Include the 5 *W*'s in your calendar or planner:
  - *Who*
  - *What* is it for
  - *What* do you need
  - *When*
  - *Where*.
- Use simple lists for simple tasks.
- Use the four-quadrant system for projects:
  - Important/urgent
  - Important/not urgent
  - Not important/urgent
  - Not important/not urgent.
- Use reminders.
- Use a pillbox.

IMPROVE YOUR PROCEDURAL MEMORY SKILLS

- Don't develop bad habits: *Take lessons.*
- Practice, practice, practice.
- Use feedback to improve your practice and your performance.
- Work with a teacher or coach.
- Space out your practice to optimize offline learning.
- Minimize interference; don't practice a competing skill.
- Start easy, build up slowly, and challenge yourself.
- Vary your practice and perform under a variety of conditions.

BASIC EPISODIC MEMORY STRATEGIES

- Strategies when acquiring memories
  - Be motivated.
  - Align your in-the-moment goals with your memory goals.
  - Relax; don't be anxious.
  - Use effort to do **FOUR** things:
    - **Focus** attention: Be present, pay attention. Avoid distraction—don't multitask. Take breaks when needed. Consider a cup of coffee (or tea). Use your sensations. Create sensational mnemonics.
    - **Organize** and cluster: Chunk that information. Make acronyms.
    - **Understand**, and generate content yourself to test your understanding. Build from the foundations up.
    - **Relate**: Make associations. Create visual images.
  - Take ownership of your learning.
  - Make it distinctive: *Involve the senses. Use humor. Imbue it with emotion. Make it important to you.*
  - Acquire content in the way you will need to retrieve it.
  - Choose whether you will remember or forget it.
  - Beware of illusions of mastery.
  - Test yourself.
  - Space out your studying—avoid cramming.
  - Vary your studying.

- ○ Interleave your studying.
- ○ Study under different conditions.
- ○ Solve the problem first, then learn how to do it.
- Strategies when retrieving memories
  - ○ Stay calm: Let your body relax; breathe deeply.
  - ○ Minimize interference and blocking: *Avoid generating possible alternatives to the right answer.*
  - ○ Create general and diverse retrieval cues.
  - ○ Return mentally to the internal and external context of your learning.
  - ○ Protect against false memories: *Evaluate the details. Could it have happened that way? How well should you remember this content?*
  - ○ Did you use extra effort? That will help for next time!
- Match your learning to the nature of what is being taught. *Learn visually and auditorily whenever possible.*
- Study together—and alone.
- Use sleep as a strategy.
- Reflect upon your retrieval.

REMEMBER NAMES

- To learn names:
  - ○ Pay attention.
  - ○ Spell the name.
  - ○ Repeat the name.
  - ○ Make a remark about the name.
  - ○ Make an association.
  - ○ Create an image.
  - ○ Find the facial feature.
  - ○ Connect your image to the facial feature.
  - ○ Add other connections.
  - ○ Repeat the connection.
  - ○ Effort is good and practice makes perfect.
- To retrieve names:
  - ○ Don't panic: If you can't remember a name, focus on another goal, such as being welcoming and friendly.

- ○ Minimize interference and blocking: *Don't keep saying the wrong name!*
- ○ Generate general retrieval cues.
- ○ Think of when you were with them.
- ○ Use the alphabet.
- ○ Review names ahead of time.
- ○ Still can't recall their name? Just ask them!

ADVANCED STRATEGIES AND MNEMONICS

- Use the method of loci, your memory palace.
- Use pictures to cue you.
- Chain images together.
- For lectures and speeches, chain images or use your memory palace.
- Use the phonetic number system:
  - ○ 1 = t, d, th; 2 = n; 3 = m; 4 = r; 5 = l; 6 = j, sh, ch, soft g; 7 = k, hard c, hard g, q, hard x; 8 = f, v, ph; 9 = p, b; 0 = s, soft c, z, soft x.
- Use peg lists:
  - ○ Phonetic number peg list: 0 = zoo, 1 = tie, 2 = Noah, 3 = ma, 4 = rye, 5 = law, 6 = shoe, 7 = cow, 8 = ivy, 9 = bee, 10 = toes, 11 = tide, 12 = tin, 13 = tomb, 14 = tire, 15 = tail, 16 = dish, 17 = dog, 18 = dove, 19 = tub, 20 = nose, etc.
  - ○ Rhyming peg list: 1 is bun; 2 is shoe; 3 is tree; 4 is store; 5 is hive; 6 is tricks; 7 is heaven; 8 is gate; 9 is twine; 10 is pen; 11 is penny one, setting sun; 12 is penny two, airplane glue; 13 is penny tree, bumblebee; etc.
- Use images for letters:
  - ○ A = apple, B = bee, C = cat, D = dog, E = elephant, etc.
- Remember passwords by combining the phonetic number system and images for letters.
- Use images for playing cards based on the phonetic number system.
- For directions, use images, the phonetic number system, and chaining.
- Remember: distinctive images are memorable.

Appendix

Medications that can impair memory

Note that it is important to consult your doctor prior to stopping or lowering the dose of one of your medications. In addition, dosages of some medications must be lowered slowly or complications—such as seizures—may occur.

ANTICHOLINERGIC ANTIDEPRESSANTS

Most currently prescribed antidepressants are safe with few side effects. The ones that do cause memory problems are those that are anticholinergic. Acetylcholine is an important chemical in the brain that is necessary for normal memory function. Medications that are anticholinergic disrupt the activity of this important brain chemical, impairing memory and sometimes causing drowsiness and confusion as well. Older antidepressants with prominent anticholinergic side effects include:

- Amitriptyline (Elavil, Endep)
- Amoxapine (Asendin)
- Clomipramine (Anafranil)

- Desipramine (Norpramin, Pertofrane)
- Doxepin (Adapin, Sinequan)
- Imipramine (Tofranil)
- Mirtazapine (Remeron)
- Nortriptyline (Pamelor, Aventyl)
- Paroxetine (Paxil)
- Protriptyline (Vivactil)
- Trazodone (Desyrel)
- Trimipramine (Surmontil)

ANTIHISTAMINES

Because they contain older formulations of antihistamines, many allergy medications, cold and flu remedies, nighttime pain relievers, and over-the-counter sleeping pills impair memory and cause drowsiness and confusion. Some of the older antihistamines that may impair memory include:

- Brompheniramine (Lodrane)
- Chlorpheniramine (Chlor-Trimeton, others)
- Diphenhydramine (Benadryl, others)
- Doxylamine (Unisom, others)
- Hydroxyzine (Vistaril, others)

ANTIPSYCHOTICS

Antipsychotics are medications that have been developed to treat young adults with schizophrenia or mania, although they are often prescribed for individuals with dementia with difficult behaviors. Memory impairment is common with these medications, particularly the older, so-called "typical" antipsychotics:

- Chlorpromazine (Thorazine)
- Fluphenazine (Prolixin)
- Haloperidol (Haldol)
- Loxapine (Adasuve)

- Mesoridazine (Serentil)
- Molindone (Moban)
- Perphenazine (Trilafon)
- Thioridazine (Mellaril)
- Thiothixene (Navane)
- Trifluoperazine (Stelazine)

The newer, "atypical" antipsychotics listed next are less likely to cause memory impairment, although they absolutely still can, particularly in high doses:

- Aripiprazole (Abilify)
- Asenapine (Saphris, Sycrest)
- Brexpiprazole (Rexulti)
- Cariprazine (Reagila)
- Clozapine (Clozaril)
- Iloperidone (Fanapt)
- Lurasidone (Latuda)
- Olanzapine (Zyprexa)
- Paliperidone (Invega)
- Pimavanserin (Nuplazid)
- Quetiapine (Seroquel)
- Risperidone (Risperdal)
- Ziprasidone (Geodon)

ANXIETY MEDICATIONS: BENZODIAZEPINES

Benzodiazepines are one class of medications used to treat anxiety that almost always causes memory impairment, drowsiness, and confusion. In fact, when doctors perform a medical procedure but don't want you to remember it (such as a colonoscopy), this is the class of medication they give you. Note that any reduction or stopping of these medications should always be done under the supervision of your doctor; seizures may occur if they are stopped abruptly. Some commonly prescribed benzodiazepines, all of which cause memory impairment, are:

- Alprazolam (Xanax)
- Chlordiazepoxide (Librium)
- Clobazam (Onfi)
- Clonazepam (Klonopin)
- Clorazepate (Tranxene)
- Diazepam (Valium)
- Estazolam (Prosom)
- Flurazepam (Dalmane, Dalmadorm)
- Lorazepam (Ativan)
- Nitrazepam (Mogadon)
- Oxazepam (Serax)
- Temazepam (Restoril)
- Triazolam (Halcion)

DIZZINESS AND VERTIGO MEDICATIONS

If you experience dizziness, nausea, and vertigo due to an inner ear infection or being on a boat, it is fine to take one of these medications for a day or two if it makes you more comfortable. But you don't want to take the medications on this list for longer than that, as they are either anticholinergic, antihistamines, or benzodiazepines, which (as described earlier in this section) all cause memory impairment:

- Clonazepam (Klonopin) (benzodiazepine)
- Diazepam (Valium) (benzodiazepine)
- Dimenhydrinate (Dramamine) (anticholinergic)
- Lorazepam (Ativan) (benzodiazepine)
- Meclizine (Antivert, Vertin) (anticholinergic)
- Metoclopramide (Reglan)
- Promethazine (Phenadoz, Phenergan, Promethegan) (antihistamine)
- Scopolamine (also known as hyoscine, anticholinergic)

HERBAL REMEDIES

Herbal remedies are just another type of medication with their own side effects; they are not intrinsically safer just because they are herbal. Common herbal medications and their major side effects include:

- Ephedra (*ma huang*): insomnia, nervousness, tremor, headache, seizure, high blood pressure, heart problems, strokes, kidney stones; memory may or may not be affected
- Ginkgo biloba: bleeding (Note: There is no evidence that ginkgo biloba improves memory, and we do not recommend its use.)
- Kava: memory impairment, sedation, confusion, abnormal movements
- St. John's wort: memory impairment, fatigue, dizziness, confusion, dry mouth, stomach upset

INCONTINENCE MEDICATIONS: ANTISPASMODICS

Bladder incontinence leading to urinary accidents is a serious problem that may make it difficult for people to go out in public and may result in wearing adult absorbent undergarments. If you or a loved one have incontinence and are taking a medication that works to stop or greatly diminish accidents, we recommend continuing it. However, many people take incontinence medications without a noticeable reduction in accidents. If this is the case, and it is one of the anticholinergic medications listed here, we recommend speaking with the doctor to see if it can be reduced, eliminated, or replaced with one that works as well or better with fewer side effects:

- Darifenacin (Enablex)
- Fesoterodine (Toviaz)
- Flavoxate (Urispas)

- Oxybutynin (Ditropan)
- Solifenacin (Vesicare)
- Tolterodine (Detrol)
- Trospium (Sanctura) (may have relatively fewer side effects)

MIGRAINE MEDICATIONS

Not all migraine medications cause memory impairment, but some do. If you are frequently taking one of the medications on this list, consider speaking with your doctor about trying a migraine medication that is less likely to cause memory impairment.

Anticholinergic Antidepressants
- Amitriptyline (Elavil, Endep)
- Doxepin (Adapin, Sinequan)
- Imipramine (Tofranil)
- Nortriptyline (Pamelor, Aventyl)
- Protriptyline (Vivactil)

Butalbital-Containing Medications
- Butalbital–acetaminophen–caffeine (Fioricet, Vanatol LQ, Vanatol S, Esgic, Capacet, and Zebutal)
- Butalbital–aspirin–caffeine (Fiorinal)

Narcotics
- Codeine–acetaminophen (Tylenol–Codeine #3)
- Oxycodone–acetaminophen (Percocet)

Seizure Medications
- Divalproex sodium (valproic acid and sodium valproate) (Depakote)
- Gabapentin (Neurontin)
- Topiramate (Topamax)

MUSCLE RELAXANTS

Medications to treat muscle spasms may be effective, but many also cause memory impairment, drowsiness, and confusion, such as:

- Baclofen (Lioresal)
- Carisoprodol (Soma)
- Chlorzoxazone (Lorzone)
- Cyclobenzaprine (Flexeril)
- Metaxalone (Skelaxin) (may have relatively fewer side effects)
- Methocarbamol (Robaxin) (may have relatively fewer side effects)
- Orphenadrine (Norflex) (anticholinergic)
- Oxazepam (Serax) (benzodiazepine)
- Tizanidine (Zanaflex)

NARCOTICS: OPIOIDS

Sometimes narcotic pain medications are needed. By itself, pain will impair memory. However, narcotics should only be used for brief periods of time. Studies have shown that they tend not to work for chronic pain, cause memory impairment and confusion, and are quite addictive. Narcotics likely to cause memory impairment include:

- Alfentanil
- Buprenorphine (Belbuca, Probuphine, Buprenex)
- Codeine (in Tylenol–Codeine #3 and some cough syrups)
- Fentanyl (Actiq, Duragesic, Fentora, Abstral, Onsolis)
- Hydrocodone (Hysingla, Zohydro, in Vicodin, Lorcet, others)
- Hydromorphone (Dilaudid, Exalgo)
- Levorphanol (Levo-Dromoran)
- Meperidine (Demerol)
- Methadone (Dolophine, Methadose)
- Morphine (MS Contin, Kadian, Morphabond)
- Nalbuphine (Nalbuphine)

- Opium
- Oxycodone (OxyContin, Oxaydo in Percocet, Roxicet)
- Oxymorphone (Opana)
- Pentazocine (Talwin)
- Propoxyphene (Darvon)
- Remifentanil (Ultiva)
- Sufentanil (Dsuvia, Sufenta)
- Tapentadol (Nucynta)
- Tramadol (ConZip, Ultram)

NAUSEA, STOMACH, AND BOWEL MEDICATIONS

Most gastrointestinal medications do not cause memory problems, but the ones listed here do:

- Chlordiazepoxide (Librium) (benzodiazepine)
- Clidinium (Librax) (anticholinergic)
- Dicyclomine (Bentyl) (anticholinergic)
- Diphenhydramine (Benadryl, others) (antihistamine)
- Glycopyrrolate (Cuvposa, Glycate, Robinul) (anticholinergic)
- Haloperidol (Haldol) (antipsychotic)
- Hyoscyamine (also known as scopolamine) (Levsin, Hyosyne, Oscimin) (anticholinergic)
- Lorazepam (Ativan) (benzodiazepine)
- Methylscopolamine (Extendryl, AlleRx, Rescon, Pamine) (anticholinergic)
- Metoclopramide (Reglan)
- Prochlorperazine (Compro) (antipsychotic)
- Propantheline (Pro-Banthine) (anticholinergic)

SEIZURE MEDICATIONS: ANTICONVULSANTS

Anticonvulsants are prescribed not only for seizures but also for nerve pain, peripheral neuropathy, headaches, mood stabilization, and agitation. Some of the anticonvulsants that can cause memory impairment include:

- Clobazam (Onfi) (benzodiazepine)
- Clonazepam (Klonopin) (benzodiazepine)
- Diazepam (Valium) (benzodiazepine)
- Divalproex sodium (Depakote)
- Gabapentin (Neurontin) (side effects may be tolerable when used in low doses [100 to 300 mg per day])
- Lorazepam (Ativan) (benzodiazepine)
- Nitrazepam (Mogadon) (benzodiazepine)
- Phenobarbital
- Phenytoin (Dilantin)
- Pregabalin (Lyrica)
- Primidone (Mysoline)
- Sodium valproate (Depakote)
- Tiagabine (Gabitril)
- Topiramate (Trokendi, Qudexy, Topamax)
- Valproic acid (Depakote)
- Vigabatrin (Sabril)

SLEEPING MEDICATIONS

Melatonin and acetaminophen are two medications that can sometimes be helpful for sleep. Otherwise, as discussed in Chapter 20, we recommend nonpharmacological treatments for sleep problems. Medications used for sleep problems that are likely to cause memory impairment and confusion the next day include:

- Amitriptyline (Elavil, Endep) (antidepressants)
- Clonazepam (Klonopin) (benzodiazepine)
- Diphenhydramine (Benadryl, in Advil PM, Tylenol PM, others) (see the earlier section on antihistamines)
- Doxepin (Adapin, Sinequan) (anticholinergic antidepressant)
- Estazolam (Prosom) (benzodiazepine)

- Eszopiclone (Lunesta) (similar to benzodiazepines)
- Flurazepam (Dalmane, Dalmadorm) (benzodiazepine)
- Gabapentin (Neurontin) (anticonvulsant)
- Lorazepam (Ativan) (benzodiazepine)
- Mirtazapine (Remeron) (anticholinergic antidepressant)
- Quetiapine (Seroquel) (antipsychotic)
- Ramelteon (Rozerem) (similar to benzodiazepines)
- Suvorexant (Belsomra) (similar to benzodiazepines)
- Temazepam (Restoril) (benzodiazepine)
- Trazodone (Desyrel) (anticholinergic antidepressant)
- Triazolam (Halcion) (benzodiazepine)
- Zaleplon (Sonata) (similar to benzodiazepines)
- Zolpidem (Ambien, ZolpiMist) (similar to benzodiazepines)

TREMOR MEDICATIONS

Tremor medications likely to cause memory impairment, drowsiness, and confusion include:

- Benztropine (Cogentin) (anticholinergic)
- Hyoscyamine (Levsin, Hyosyne, Oscimin) (anticholinergic)
- Primidone (Mysoline) (anticonvulsant)
- Trihexyphenidyl (Artane) (anticholinergic)

References

PREFACE

1. Simons, D. J., & Chabris, C. F. (2011). What people believe about how memory works: A representative survey of the U.S. population. *PloS One*, *6*(8), e22757. https://doi.org/10.1371/journal.pone.0022757

CHAPTER 1: MEMORY IS NOT ONE THING

1. Scoville, W. B., & Milner, B. (1957). Loss of recent memory after bilateral hippocampal lesions. *Journal of Neurology, Neurosurgery, and Psychiatry*, *20*(1), 11–21. https://doi.org/10.1136/jnnp.20.1.11
2. Skotko, B. G., Kensinger, E. A., Locascio, J. J., Einstein, G., Rubin, D. C., Tupler, L. A., Krendl, A., & Corkin, S. (2004). Puzzling thoughts for H. M.: Can new semantic information be anchored to old semantic memories?. *Neuropsychology*, *18*(4), 756–769. https://doi.org/10.1037/0894-4105.18.4.756
3. Kensinger, E. A., Ullman, M. T., & Corkin, S. (2001). Bilateral medial temporal lobe damage does not affect lexical or grammatical processing: Evidence from amnesic patient H.M. *Hippocampus*, *11*(4), 347–360. https://doi.org/10.1002/hipo.1049

4. Bohbot, V. D., & Corkin, S. (2007). Posterior parahippocampal place learning in H.M. *Hippocampus, 17*(9), 863–872. https://doi.org/10.1002/hipo.20313

CHAPTER 2: MUSCLE MEMORY

1. Macnamara, B. N., Moreau, D., & Hambrick, D. Z. (2016). The relationship between deliberate practice and performance in sports: A meta-analysis. *Perspectives on Psychological Science, 11*(3), 333–350. https://doi.org/10.1177/1745691616635591
2. Baddeley, A. D., & Longman, D. (1978). The influence of length and frequency of training session on the rate of learning to type. *Ergonomics, 21,* 627–635.
3. Robertson, E. M., Press, D. Z., & Pascual-Leone, A. (2005). Off-line learning and the primary motor cortex. *Journal of Neuroscience, 25*(27), 6372–6378. https://doi.org/10.1523/JNEUROSCI.1851-05.2005
4. Fox, P. W., Hershberger, S. L., & Bouchard, T. J., Jr. (1996). Genetic and environmental contributions to the acquisition of a motor skill. *Nature, 384,* 356–358.
5. Vakil, E., Kahan, S., Huberman, M., & Osimani, A. (2000). Motor and non-motor sequence learning in patients with basal ganglia lesions: The case of serial reaction time (SRT). *Neuropsychologia, 38*(1), 1–10. https://doi.org/10.1016/s0028-3932(99)00058-5
6. Poldrack, R. A., Clark, J., Paré-Blagoev, E. J., Shohamy, D., Creso Moyano, J., Myers, C., & Gluck, M. A. (2001). Interactive memory systems in the human brain. *Nature, 414*(6863), 546–550. https://doi.org/10.1038/35107080
7. Ahmadian, N., van Baarsen, K., van Zandvoort, M., & Robe, P. A. (2019). The cerebellar cognitive affective syndrome: A meta-analysis. *Cerebellum, 18*(5), 941–950. https://doi.org/10.1007/s12311-019-01060-2
8. Elbert, T., Pantev, C., Wienbruch, C., Rockstroh, B., & Taub, E. (1995). Increased cortical representation of the fingers of the left hand in string players. *Science, 270,* 305–307.

9. Tang, Y. Y., Tang, Y., Tang, R., & Lewis-Peacock, J. A. (2017). Brief mental training reorganizes large-scale brain networks. *Frontiers in Systems Neuroscience, 11*, 6. https://doi.org/10.3389/fnsys.2017.00006

CHAPTER 3: KEEP IT IN MIND

1. Miller, G. (1956). The magic number seven plus or minus two: Some limits on our capacity for processing information. *Psychological Review, 63*, 81–97.
2. Cowan, N. (2001). The magical number 4 in short-term memory: A reconsideration of mental storage capacity. *Behavioral and Brain Sciences, 24*(1), 87–185. https://doi.org/10.1017/s0140525x01003922
3. Ericsson, K. A., & Chase, W. G. (1982). Exceptional memory: Extraordinary feats of memory can be matched or surpassed by people with average memories that have been improved by training. *American Scientist, 70*(6), 607–615. http://www.jstor.org/stable/27851732
4. Repovs, G., & Baddeley, A. (2006). The multi-component model of working memory: Explorations in experimental cognitive psychology. *Neuroscience, 139*(1), 5–21. https://doi.org/10.1016/j.neuroscience.2005.12.061
5. Mazoyer, B., Zago, L., Jobard, G., Crivello, F., Joliot, M., Perchey, G., Mellet, E., Petit, L., & Tzourio-Mazoyer, N. (2014). Gaussian mixture modeling of hemispheric lateralization for language in a large sample of healthy individuals balanced for handedness. *PloS One, 9*(6), e101165. https://doi.org/10.1371/journal.pone.0101165
6. Badre, D. (2008). Cognitive control, hierarchy, and the rostro-caudal organization of the frontal lobes. *Trends in Cognitive Sciences, 12*, 193–200.
7. Shaw, P., Kabani, N. J., Lerch, J. P., Eckstrand, K., Lenroot, R., Gogtay, N., Greenstein, D., Clasen, L., Evans, A., Rapoport, J. L., Giedd, J. N., & Wise, S. P. (2008). Neurodevelopmental trajectories of the human cerebral cortex. *Journal of Neuroscience, 28*, 3586–3594.

CHAPTER 4: TRAVEL BACK IN TIME

1. Ribot, T. (1882). *The diseases of memory.* Appleton.
2. Ally, B. A., Simons, J. S., McKeever, J. D., Peers, P. V., & Budson, A. E. (2008). Parietal contributions to recollection: Electrophysiological evidence from aging and patients with parietal lesions. *Neuropsychologia, 46*(7), 1800–1812. https://doi.org/10.1016/j.neuropsychologia.2008.02.026
3. Moscovitch, M., Cabeza, R., Winocur, G., & Nadel, L. (2016). Episodic memory and beyond: The hippocampus and neocortex in transformation. *Annual Review of Psychology, 67,* 105–134. https://doi.org/10.1146/annurev-psych-113011-143733

CHAPTER 5: WHAT YOU KNOW

1. Damasio, H., Grabowski, T. J., Tranel, D., Hichwa, R. D., & Damasio, A. R. (1996). A neural basis for lexical retrieval. *Nature, 380*(6574), 499–505. https://doi.org/10.1038/380499a0

CHAPTER 6: WHAT WE REMEMBER TOGETHER

1. Congleton, A. R., & Rajaram, S. (2014). Collaboration changes both the content and the structure of memory: Building the architecture of shared representations. *Journal of Experimental Psychology: General, 143*(4), 1570–1584.
2. Roediger, H. L., & DeSoto, A. (2016). The power of collective memory. *Scientific American.* https://www.scientificameri can.com/article/the-power-of-collective-memory/
3. Gokhale, A. A. (1995). Collaborative learning enhances critical thinking. *Journal of Technology Education, 7*(1). https://doi.org/10.21061/jte.v7i1.a.2
4. Rajaram, S. (2011). Collaboration both hurts and helps memory: A cognitive perspective. *Current Directions*

in Psychological Science, *20*(2), 76–81. doi:10.1177/ 0963721411403251

5. Speer, M. E., Bhanji, J. P., & Delgado, M. R. (2014). Savoring the past: Positive memories evoke value representations in the striatum. *Neuron, 84*(4), 847–856. https://doi.org/10.1016/ j.neuron.2014.09.028

6. Sheen, M., Kemp, S., & Rubin, D. (2001). Twins dispute memory ownership: A new false memory phenomenon. *Memory & Cognition, 29*, 779–788.

7. French, L., Gerrie, M. P., Garry, M., & Mori, K. (2009). Evidence for the efficacy of the MORI technique: Viewers do not notice or implicitly remember details from the alternate movie version. *Behavior Research Methods, 41*(4), 1224–1232. https://doi.org/10.3758/BRM.41.4.1224

CHAPTER 7: DO YOU NEED TO TRY TO REMEMBER?

1. Tulving, E. (1972). Episodic and semantic memory. In E. Tulving, & W. Donaldson (Eds.), *Organization of memory* (pp. 381–403). Academic Press.

2. Renoult, L., & Rugg, M.D. (2020). An historical perspective on Endel Tulving's episodic-semantic distinction. *Neuropsychologia, 139.* https://doi.org/10.1016/j.neuropsychologia.2020.107366

3. Nickerson, R. S., & Adams, M. J. (1979). Long-term memory for a common object. *Cognitive Psychology, 11*(3), 287–307. https://doi.org/10.1016/0010-0285(79)90013-6

4. Brandsford, J. D. (1972). Contextual prerequisites for understanding: Some investigations of comprehension and recall. *Journal of Verbal Learning and Verbal Behavior, 11*(16), 717–726.

5. Craik, F. I. M., Govoni, R., Naveh-Benjamin, M., & Anderson, N. D. (1996). The effects of divided attention on

encoding and retrieval processes in human memory. *Journal of Experimental Psychology: General, 125*(2), 159–180. https://doi.org/10.1037/0096-3445.125.2.159

6. Rahhal, T. A., Hasher, L., & Colcombe, S. J. (2001). Instructional manipulations and age differences in memory: Now you see them, now you don't. *Psychology and Aging, 16*(4), 697–706. https://doi.org/10.1037/0882-7974.16.4.697

CHAPTER 8: GET IT INTO YOUR MEMORY— AND KEEP IT THERE

1. Oliva, A., & Torralba, A. (2006). Building the gist of a scene: The role of global image features in recognition. *Progress in Brain Research, 155,* 23–36. https://doi.org/10.1016/S0079-6123(06)55002-2

2. Gobet, F. (1998). Expert memory: A comparison of four theories. *Cognition, 66*(2), 115–152. https://doi.org/10.1016/s0010-0277(98)00020-1

3. Ebbinghaus, H. (1885). *Memory: A contribution to experimental psychology.* New York by Teachers College, Columbia University. Translated by Henry A. Ruger & Clara E. Bussenius (1913). http://psychclassics.yorku.ca/Ebbinghaus/index.htm

4. Schacter, D. L. (2001, May 1). The seven sins of memory. *Psychology Today.* https://www.psychologytoday.com/us/articles/200105/the-seven-sins-memory

5. Cooper, R. A., Kensinger, E. A., & Ritchey, M. (2019). Memories fade: The relationship between memory vividness and remembered visual salience. *Psychological Science, 30*(5), 657–668. https://doi.org/10.1177/0956797619836093

6. Richter-Levin, G., & Akirav, I. (2003). Emotional tagging of memory formation—in the search for neural mechanisms. *Brain Research Reviews, 43*(3), 247–256. https://doi.org/10.1016/j.brainrev.2003.08.005

7. Hunt, R. R., & Worthen, J. B. (Eds.). (2006). *Distinctiveness and memory.* Oxford University Press. https://doi.org/10.1093/acprof:oso/9780195169669.001.0001

8. MacLeod, C. M., Gopie, N., Hourihan, K. L., Neary, K. R., & Ozubko, J. D. (2010). The production effect: Delineation of a phenomenon. *Journal of Experimental Psychology: Learning, Memory, and Cognition, 36*(3), 671–685. https://doi.org/10.1037/a0018785

9. The benefits of forgetting were espoused by the philosopher William James in *The Principles of Psychology,* when he wrote, "In the practical use of our intellect, forgetting is as important a function as remembering." And these benefits have continued to be supported by scientific research (https://media.nature.com/original/magazine-assets/d41586-019-02211-5/d41586-019-02211-5.pdf).

10. Schacter, D. L., Addis, D. R., & Buckner, R. L. (2007). Remembering the past to imagine the future: The prospective brain. *Nature Reviews Neuroscience, 8*(9), 657–661. https://doi.org/10.1038/nrn2213

CHAPTER 9: RETRIEVE THAT MEMORY

1. Josselyn, S. A., Köhler, S., & Frankland, P. W. (2017). Heroes of the Engram. *Journal of Neuroscience, 37*(18), 4647–4657. https://doi.org/10.1523/JNEUROSCI.0056-17.2017

2. Brown, R., & McNeill, D. (1966). The "tip-of-the-tongue" phenomenon. *Journal of Verbal Learning and Verbal Behavior, 5,* 325–337.

3. Conway, M. A., & Pleydell-Pearce, C. W. (2000). The construction of autobiographical memories in the self-memory system. *Psychological Review, 107*(2), 261–288. https://doi.org/10.1037/0033-295x.107.2.261

4. Nadel, L., & Moscovitch, M. (1997). Memory consolidation, retrograde amnesia and the hippocampal complex. *Current*

Opinion in Neurobiology, 7, 217–227. https://doi.org/10.1016/S0959-4388(97)80010-4

5. McDaniel, M. A., & Einstein, G. O. (2007). *Prospective memory: An overview and synthesis of an emerging field.* SAGE Publications, Inc. https://www.doi.org/10.4135/9781452225913

6. Godden, D. R., & Baddeley, A. D. (1975). Context-dependent memory in two natural environments: On land and underwater. *British Journal of Psychology, 66*(3), 325–331.

CHAPTER 10: ASSOCIATE INFORMATION

1. Yonelinas, A. P. (2001). Components of episodic memory: The contribution of recollection and familiarity. *Philosophical Transactions of the Royal Society of London. Series B, Biological Sciences, 356*(1413), 1363–1374. https://doi.org/10.1098/rstb.2001.0939

2. Johnson, M. K. (1997). Source monitoring and memory distortion. *Philosophical Transactions of the Royal Society of London. Series B, Biological Sciences, 352*(1362), 1733–1745. https://doi.org/10.1098/rstb.1997.0156

3. Gopie, N., & MacLeod, C. (2009). "Destination memory: Stop me if I've told you this before." *Psychological Science, 20,* 1492–1499. doi:10.1111/j.1467-9280.2009.02472.x

4. Davachi, L., & DuBrow, S. (2015). How the hippocampus preserves order: The role of prediction and context. *Trends in Cognitive Sciences, 19*(2), 92–99. https://doi.org/10.1016/j.tics.2014.12.004

5. Walker, W. R., & Skowronski, J. J. (2009). The fading affect bias: But what the hell is it for? *Applied Cognitive Psychology, 23*(8), 1122–1136. https://doi.org/10.1002/acp.1614

6. Kensinger, E. A., Garoff-Eaton, R. J., & Schacter, D. L. (2007). Effects of emotion on memory specificity: Memory trade-offs elicited by negative visually arousing stimuli. *Journal of*

Memory and Language, 56, 575–591. https://doi.org/10.1016/j.jml.2006.05.004

7. Schlichting, M. L., & Preston, A. R. (2015). Memory integration: Neural mechanisms and implications for behavior. *Current Opinion in Behavioral Sciences, 1*, 1–8. https://doi.org/10.1016/j.cobeha.2014.07.005

CHAPTER 11: CONTROL WHAT YOU FORGET AND REMEMBER

1. Dunsmoor, J. E., Murty, V. P., Davachi, L., & Phelps, E. A. (2015). Emotional learning selectively and retroactively strengthens episodic memories for related events. *Nature, 520*, 345–348.

2. Bjork, R. A. (1989). Retrieval inhibition as an adaptive mechanism in human memory. In H. L. Roediger & F. I. M. Craik (Eds.), *Varieties of memory and consciousness: Essays in honour of Endel Tulving* (pp. 309–330). Erlbaum.

3. Guillory, J. J., & Geraci, L. (2016). The persistence of erroneous information in memory: The effect of valence on the acceptance of corrected information. *Applied Cognitive Psychology, 30*(2), 282–288. https://doi.org/10.1002/acp.3183

4. Wegner, D. M. (1987). Transactive memory: A contemporary analysis of the group mind. In B. Mullen & G. R. Goethals (Eds.), *Theories of group behavior* (pp. 185–208). Springer Series in Social Psychology. Springer. https://doi.org/10.1007/978-1-4612-4634-3_9

5. Jackson, M., & Moreland, R. L. (2009). Transactive memory in the classroom. *Small Group Research, 40*(5), 508–534. https://doi.org/10.1177/1046496409340703

6. Gagnepain, P., Hulbert, J., & Anderson, M. C. (2017). Parallel regulation of memory and emotion supports the suppression of intrusive memories. *Journal of Neuroscience, 37*(27), 6423–6441. https://doi.org/10.1523/JNEUROSCI.2732-16.2017

7. Anderson, M. C., & Hanslmayr, S. (2014). Neural mechanisms of motivated forgetting. *Trends in Cognitive Sciences, 18*(6), 279–292. https://doi.org/10.1016/j.tics.2014.03.002

CHAPTER 12: ARE YOU SURE THAT'S NOT A FALSE MEMORY?

1. Wixted, J. T., & Wells, G. L. (2017). The relationship between eyewitness confidence and identification accuracy: A new synthesis. *Psychological Science in the Public Interest, 18*(1), 10–65. https://doi.org/10.1177/1529100616686966

2. Wade, K. A., Garry, M., Don Read, J., & Lindsay, D. S. (2002). A picture is worth a thousand lies: Using false photographs to create false childhood memories. *Psychonomic Bulletin & Review, 9*, 597–603. https://doi.org/10.3758/BF03196318

3. Steblay, N. K., Wells, G. L., & Douglass, A. B. (2014). The eyewitness post identification feedback effect 15 years later: Theoretical and policy implications. *Psychology, Public Policy, and Law, 20*(1), 1–18. https://doi.org/10.1037/law0000001

4. Loftus, E. F., & Hoffman, H. G. (1989). Misinformation and memory: The creation of new memories. *Journal of Experimental Psychology: General, 118*(1), 100–104. https://doi.org/10.1037/0096-3445.118.1.100

5. Loftus, E. F., Miller, D. G., & Burns, H. J. (1978). Semantic integration of verbal information into a visual memory. *Journal of Experimental Psychology: Human Learning and Memory, 4*(1), 19–31. https://doi.org/10.1037/0278-7393.4.1.19

6. Otgaar, H., Romeo, T., Ramakers, N., & Howe, M. L. (2018). Forgetting having denied: The "amnesic" consequences of denial. *Memory & Cognition, 46*(4), 520–529. https://doi.org/10.3758/s13421-017-0781-5

7. Roediger, H. L., & McDermott, K. B. (1995). Creating false memories: Remembering words not presented in lists.

Journal of Experimental Psychology: Learning, Memory, and Cognition, *21*(4), 803–814. https://doi.org/10.1037/0278-7393.21.4.803

8. Mitchell, J. P., Sullivan, A. L., Schacter, D. L., & Budson, A. E. (2006). Mis-attribution errors in Alzheimer's disease: The illusory truth effect. *Neuropsychology, 20*(2), 185–192. https://doi.org/10.1037/0894-4105.20.2.185

9. Brown, R., & Kulik, J. (1977). Flashbulb memories. *Cognition, 5*, 73–99.

10. Neisser, U., & Harsch, N. (1992). Phantom flashbulbs: False recollections of hearing the news about Challenger. In E. Winograd & U. Neisser (Eds.), *Emory symposia in cognition, 4. Affect and accuracy in recall: Studies of "flashbulb" memories* (pp. 9–31). Cambridge University Press. https://doi.org/10.1017/CBO9780511664069.003

11. Talarico, J. M., & Rubin, D. C. (2003). Confidence, not consistency, characterizes flashbulb memories. *Psychological Science, 14*(5), 455–461. https://doi.org/10.1111/1467-9280.02453

12. Paller, K. A., Antony, J. W., Mayes, A. R., & Norman, K. A. (2020). Replay-based consolidation governs enduring memory storage. In D. Poeppel, G. R. Mangun, & M.S. Gazzaniga (Eds.), *The cognitive neurosciences* (6th ed.). MIT Press.

13. Loftus, E. F., Loftus, G. R., & Messo, J. (1987). Some facts about "weapon focus." *Law and Human Behavior, 11*(1), 55–62. https://doi.org/10.1007/BF01044839

14. Steinmetz, K. R., & Kensinger, E. A. (2013). The emotion-induced memory trade-off: More than an effect of overt attention? *Memory & Cognition, 41*(1), 69–81. https://doi.org/10.3758/s13421-012-0247-8

15. Rotello, C. M., & Heit, E. (1999). Two-process models of recognition memory: Evidence for recall-to-reject? *Journal of Memory and Language, 40*(3), 432–453. https://doi.org/10.1006/jmla.1998.2623

CHAPTER 13: JUST NORMAL AGING—OR IS IT ALZHEIMER'S DISEASE?

1. Alzheimer, A., Stelzmann, R. A., Schnitzlein, H. N., & Murtagh, F. R. (1995). An English translation of Alzheimer's 1907 paper, "Uber eine eigenartige Erkankung der Hirnrinde." *Clinical Anatomy, 8*(6), 429–431. https://doi.org/10.1002/ca.980080612
2. Budson, A. E., & O'Connor, M. K. (2023). *Seven Steps to Managing Your Aging Memory: What's Normal, What's Not, and What to Do About It.* New York: Oxford University Press.
3. Budson, A. E., & O'Connor, M. K. (2022). *Six Steps to Managing Alzheimer's Disease and Dementia: A Guide for Families.* New York: Oxford University Press.

CHAPTER 14: WHAT ELSE CAN GO WRONG WITH YOUR MEMORY?

1. Wada, H., Inagaki, N., Yamatodani, A., & Watanabe, T. (1991). Is the histaminergic neuron system a regulatory center for whole-brain activity? *Trends in Neurosciences, 14*(9), 415–418. https://doi.org/10.1016/0166-2236(91)90034-r
2. Passani, M. B., Benetti, F., Blandina, P., Furini, C., de Carvalho Myskiw, J., & Izquierdo, I. (2017). Histamine regulates memory consolidation. *Neurobiology of Learning and Memory, 145*, 1–6. https://doi.org/10.1016/j.nlm.2017.08.007
3. Zhou, H., Lu, S., Chen, J., Wei, N., Wang, D., Lyu, H., Shi, C., & Hu, S. (2020). The landscape of cognitive function in recovered COVID-19 patients. *Journal of Psychiatric Research, 129*, 98–102. https://doi.org/10.1016/j.jpsychires.2020.06.022
4. Heneka, M. T., Golenbock, D., Latz, E., Morgan, D., & Brown, R. (2020). Immediate and long-term consequences of COVID-19 infections for the development of neurological disease. *Alzheimer's Research & Therapy, 12*(1), 69. https://doi.org/10.1186/s13195-020-00640-3

5. Luo, Y., Weibman, D., Halperin, J. M., & Li, X. (2019). A review of heterogeneity in attention-deficit/hyperactivity disorder (ADHD). *Frontiers in Human Neuroscience, 13,* 42. doi:10.3389/fnhum.2019.00042

6. Kraguljac, N. V., Srivastava, A., & Lahti, A. C. (2013). Memory deficits in schizophrenia: A selective review of functional magnetic resonance imaging (FMRI) studies. *Behavioral Sciences, 3*(3), 330–347. https://doi.org/10.3390/bs3030330

7. Blomberg, M. O., Semkovska, M., Kessler, U., Erchinger, V. J., Oedegaard, K. J., Oltedal, L., & Hammar, Å. (2020). A longitudinal comparison between depressed patients receiving electroconvulsive therapy and healthy controls on specific memory functions. *Primary Care Companion for CNS Disorders, 22*(3), 19m02547. https://doi.org/10.4088/PCC.19m02547

CHAPTER 15: POST-TRAUMATIC STRESS DISORDER: WHEN YOU CAN'T FORGET

1. McKinnon, M. C., Palombo, D. J., Nazarov, A., Kumar, N., Khuu, W., & Levine, B. (2015). Threat of death and autobiographical memory: A study of passengers from Flight AT236. *Clinical Psychological Science, 3*(4), 487–502. https://doi.org/10.1177/2167702614542280

2. Brewin, C. R. (2018). Memory and forgetting. *Current Psychiatry Reports, 20*(10), 87. https://doi.org/10.1007/s11920-018-0950-7

3. Brewin, C. R., Gregory, J. D., Lipton, M., & Burgess, N. (2010). Intrusive images in psychological disorders: Characteristics, neural mechanisms, and treatment implications. *Psychological Review, 117*(1), 210–232. https://doi.org/10.1037/a0018113

4. Mayou, R., Bryant, B., & Duthie, R. (1993). Psychiatric consequences of road traffic accidents. *BMJ (Clinical Research*

Edition), *307*(6905), 647–651. https://doi.org/10.1136/bmj.307.6905.647

5. Benjet, C., Bromet, E., Karam, E. G., Kessler, R. C., McLaughlin, K. A., Ruscio, A. M., Shahly, V., Stein, D. J., Petukhova, M., Hill, E., Alonso, J., Atwoli, L., Bunting, B., Bruffaerts, R., Caldas-de-Almeida, J. M., de Girolamo, G., Florescu, S., Gureje, O., Huang, Y., Lepine, J. P., . . . Koenen, K. C. (2016). The epidemiology of traumatic event exposure worldwide: Results from the World Mental Health Survey Consortium. *Psychological Medicine*, *46*(2), 327–343. https://doi.org/10.1017/S003329171 5001981

6. Berntsen, D. (2021). Involuntary autobiographical memories and their relation to other forms of spontaneous thoughts. *Philosophical Transactions of the Royal Society of London. Series B, Biological Sciences*, *376*(1817), 20190693. https://doi.org/10.1098/rstb.2019.0693

7. Catarino, A., Küpper, C. S., Werner-Seidler, A., Dalgleish, T., & Anderson, M. C. (2015). Failing to forget: Inhibitory-control deficits compromise memory suppression in post-traumatic stress disorder. *Psychological Science*, *26*(5), 604–616. https://doi.org/10.1177/0956797615569889

8. Anderson, M. C., & Green, C. (2001). Suppressing unwanted memories by executive control. *Nature*, *410*(6826), 366–369. https://doi.org/10.1038/35066572

9. McNally, R. J., Metzger, L. J., Lasko, N. B., Clancy, S. A., & Pitman, R. K. (1998). Directed forgetting of trauma cues in adult survivors of childhood sexual abuse with and without posttraumatic stress disorder. *Journal of Abnormal Psychology*, *107*(4), 596–601. https://doi.org/10.1037//0021-843x.107.4.596

10. Reisman, M. (2016). PTSD treatment for veterans: What's working, what's new, and what's next. *Pharmacy & Therapeutics*, *41*(10), 623–634.

11. Gradus, J. L. Epidemiology of PTSD. National Center for PTSD. https://www.ptsd.va.gov/professional/treat/essenti als/epidemiology.asp

12. Neylan, T. C., Marmar, C. R., Metzler, T. J., Weiss, D. S., Zatzick, D. F., Delucchi, K. L., Wu, R. M., & Schoenfeld, F. B. (1998). Sleep disturbances in the Vietnam generation: Findings from a nationally representative sample of male Vietnam veterans. *American Journal of Psychiatry*, *155*(7), 929–933.

13. Wang, C., Laxminarayan, S., Ramakrishnan, S., Dovzhenok, A., Cashmere, J. D., Germain, A., & Reifman, J. (2020). Increased oscillatory frequency of sleep spindles in combat-exposed veteran men with post-traumatic stress disorder. *Sleep*, *43*(10), zsaa064.

14. Logue, M. W., van Rooij, S. J. H., Dennis, E. L., Davis, S. L., Hayes, J. P., Stevens, J. S., Densmore, M., Haswell, C. C., Ipser, J., Koch, S. B. J., Korgaonkar, M., Lebois, L. A. M., Peverill, M., Baker, J. T., Boedhoe, P. S. W., Frijling, J. L., Gruber, S. A., Harpaz-Rotem, I., Jahashad, N., . . . Morey, R. A. (2018). Smaller hippocampal volume in posttraumatic stress disorder: A multisite ENIGMA-PGC study: Subcortical volumetry results from posttraumatic stress disorder consortia. *Biological Psychiatry*, *83*(3), 244–253. https://doi.org/10.1016/j.biopsych.2017.09.006

15. Kremen, W. S., Koenen, K. C., Afari, N., & Lyons M. J. (2012). Twin studies of posttraumatic stress disorder: Differentiating vulnerability factors from sequelae. *Neuropharmacology*, *62*(2), 647–653. doi:10.1016/j.neuropharm.2011.03.012

16. Brewin, C. R. (2014). Episodic memory, perceptual memory, and their interaction: Foundations for a theory of posttraumatic stress disorder. *Psychological Bulletin*, *140*(1), 69–97. https://doi.org/10.1037/a0033722

17. Iyadurai, L., Visser, R. M., Lau-Zhu, A., Porcheret, K., Horsch, A., Holmes, E. A., & James, E. L. (2019). Intrusive memories of trauma: A target for research bridging cognitive science and its clinical application. *Clinical Psychology Review*, *69*, 67–82. https://doi.org/10.1016/j.cpr.2018.08.005

18. Rubin, D. C., Berntsen, D., & Bohni, M. K. (2008). A memory-based model of posttraumatic stress disorder: Evaluating

basic assumptions underlying the PTSD diagnosis. *Psychological Review, 115*(4), 985–1011. https://doi.org/10.1037/a0013397

CHAPTER 16: THOSE WHO REMEMBER EVERYTHING

1. McGaugh, J. L. (2017). Highly superior autobiographical memory. In J. H. Byrne (Ed.), *Learning and memory: A comprehensive reference* (2nd ed., Chapter 2.08). Academic Press.
2. Klüver, H. (1928). Studies on the eidetic type and on eidetic imagery. *Psychological Bulletin, 25*(2), 69–104. https://doi.org/10.1037/h0070849
3. Giray, E. F., Altkin, W. M., Vaught, G. M., & Roodin, P. A. (1976). The incidence of eidetic imagery as a function of age. *Child Development, 47*(4), 1207–1210. PMID: 1001094.
4. Frey, P. W., & Adesman, P. (1976). Recall memory for visually presented chess positions. *Memory & Cognition, 4,* 541–547.
5. Symons, C. S., & Johnson, B. T. (1997). The self-reference effect in memory: A meta-analysis. *Psychological Bulletin, 121*(3), 371–394. doi:10.1037/0033-2909.121.3.371
6. Patihis, L., Frenda, S. J., LePort, A. K., Petersen, N., Nichols, R. M., Stark, C. E., McGaugh, J. L., & Loftus, E. F. (2013). False memories in highly superior autobiographical memory individuals. *Proceedings of the National Academy of Sciences of the United States of America, 110*(52), 20947–20952. https://doi.org/10.1073/pnas.1314373110
7. Boddaert, N., Barthélémy, C., Poline, J., Samson, Y., Brunelle, F., & Zilbovicius, M. (2005). Autism: Functional brain mapping of exceptional calendar capacity. *British Journal of Psychiatry, 187*(1), 83–86. doi:10.1192/bjp.187.1.83
8. Cowan, R., & Frith, C. (2009). Do calendrical savants use calculation to answer date questions? A functional magnetic resonance imaging study. *Philosophical Transactions*

of the Royal Society of London. Series B, Biological Sciences, *364*(1522), 1417–1424. https://doi.org/10.1098/rstb.2008.0323

9. Olson, I. R., Berryhill, M. E., Drowos, D. B., Brown, L., & Chatterjee, A. (2010). A calendar savant with episodic memory impairments. *Neurocase, 16*(3), 208–218. https://doi.org/10.1080/13554790903405701

10. Kennedy, D. P., & Squire, L. R. (2007). An analysis of calendar performance in two autistic calendar savants. *Learning & Memory, 14*(8), 533–538. https://doi.org/10.1101/lm.653607

11. Libero, L. E., DeRamus, T. P., Lahti, A. C., Deshpande, G., & Kana, R. K. (2015). Multimodal neuroimaging based classification of autism spectrum disorder using anatomical, neurochemical, and white matter correlates. *Cortex, 66,* 46–59. https://doi.org/10.1016/j.cortex.2015.02.008

12. Ally, B. A., Hussey, E. P., & Donahue, M. J. (2013). A case of hyperthymesia: Rethinking the role of the amygdala in autobiographical memory. *Neurocase, 19*(2), 166–181. https://doi.org/10.1080/13554794.2011.654225

13. LePort, A. K., Mattfeld, A. T., Dickinson-Anson, H., Fallon, J. H., Stark, C. E., Kruggel, F., Cahill, L., & McGaugh, J. L. (2012). Behavioral and neuroanatomical investigation of highly superior autobiographical memory (HSAM). *Neurobiology of Learning and Memory, 98*(1), 78–92. https://doi.org/10.1016/j.nlm.2012.05.002

14. Henner, M. (2013). *Total memory makeover: Uncover your past, take charge of your future.* Gallery Books. (Quote on p. 23)

CHAPTER 17: EXERCISE: THE ELIXIR OF LIFE

1. Jadczak, A. D., Makwana, N., Luscombe-Marsh, N., Visvanathan, R., & Schultz, T. J. (2018). Effectiveness of exercise interventions on physical function in community-dwelling frail older people: An umbrella review of

systematic reviews. *JBI Database of Systematic Reviews and Implementation Reports, 16*(3), 752–775. https://doi.org/10.11124/JBISRIR-2017-003551

2. Hörder, H., Johansson, L., Guo, X., Grimby, G., Kern, S., Östling, S., & Skoog, I. (2018). Midlife cardiovascular fitness and dementia: A 44-year longitudinal population study in women. *Neurology, 90*(15), e1298–e1305. https://doi.org/10.1212/WNL.0000000000005290

3. Strazzullo, P., D'Elia, L., Cairella, G., Garbagnati, F., Cappuccio, F. P., & Scalfi, L. (2010). Excess body weight and incidence of stroke: Meta-analysis of prospective studies with 2 million participants. *Stroke, 41*(5), e418–e426. https://doi.org/10.1161/STROKEAHA.109.576967

4. Guo, Y., Yue, X. J., Li, H. H., Song, Z. X., Yan, H. Q., Zhang, P., Gui, Y. K., Chang, L., & Li, T. (2016). Overweight and obesity in young adulthood and the risk of stroke: A meta-analysis. *Journal of Stroke and Cerebrovascular Diseases, 25*(12), 2995–3004. https://doi.org/10.1016/j.jstrokecerebrovasdis.2016.08.018

5. Siebers, M., Biedermann, S. V., Bindila, L., Lutz, B., & Fuss, J. (2021). Exercise-induced euphoria and anxiolysis do not depend on endogenous opioids in humans. *Psychoneuroendocrinology, 126,* 105173. https://doi.org/10.1016/j.psyneuen.2021.105173

6. Kvam, S., Kleppe, C. L., Nordhus, I. H., & Hovland, A. (2016). Exercise as a treatment for depression: A meta-analysis. *Journal of Affective Disorders, 202,* 67–86. https://doi.org/10.1016/j.jad.2016.03.063

7. Thomas, A. G., Dennis, A., Rawlings, N. B., Stagg, C. J., Matthews, L., Morris, M., Kolind, S. H., Foxley, S., Jenkinson, M., Nichols, T. E., Dawes, H., Bandettini, P. A., & Johansen-Berg, H. (2016). Multi-modal characterization of rapid anterior hippocampal volume increase associated with aerobic exercise. *NeuroImage, 131,* 162–170. https://doi.org/10.1016/j.neuroimage.2015.10.090

8. Erickson, K. I., Voss, M. W., Prakash, R. S., Basak, C., Szabo, A., Chaddock, L., Kim, J. S., Heo, S., Alves, H., White, S. M., Wojcicki, T. R., Mailey, E., Vieira, V. J., Martin, S. A., Pence, B. D., Woods, J. A., McAuley, E., & Kramer, A. F. (2011). Exercise training increases size of hippocampus and improves memory. *Proceedings of the National Academy of Sciences of the United States of America, 108*(7), 3017–3022. https://doi.org/10.1073/pnas.1015950108

9. Liu, P. Z., & Nusslock, R. (2018). Exercise-mediated neurogenesis in the hippocampus via BDNF. *Frontiers in Neuroscience, 12*, 52. https://doi.org/10.3389/fnins.2018.00052

10. Basso, J. C., & Suzuki, W. A. (2017). The effects of acute exercise on mood, cognition, neurophysiology, and neurochemical pathways: A review. *Brain Plasticity, 2*(2), 127–152. https://doi.org/10.3233/BPL-160040

11. Smith, J. C., Nielson, K. A., Woodard, J. L., Seidenberg, M., Durgerian, S., Hazlett, K. E., Figueroa, C. M., Kandah, C. C., Kay, C. D., Matthews, M. A., & Rao, S. M. (2014). Physical activity reduces hippocampal atrophy in elders at genetic risk for Alzheimer's disease. *Frontiers in Aging Neuroscience, 6*, 61. https://doi.org/10.3389/fnagi.2014.00061

12. Morris, J. K., Vidoni, E. D., Johnson, D. K., Van Sciver, A., Mahnken, J. D., Honea, R. A., Wilkins, H. M., Brooks, W. M., Billinger, S. A., Swerdlow, R. H., & Burns, J. M. (2017). Aerobic exercise for Alzheimer's disease: A randomized controlled pilot trial. *PloS One, 12*(2), e0170547. https://doi.org/10.1371/journal.pone.0170547

13. Petersen, R. C., Lopez, O., Armstrong, M. J., Getchius, T., Ganguli, M., Gloss, D., Gronseth, G. S., Marson, D., Pringsheim, T., Day, G. S., Sager, M., Stevens, J., & Rae-Grant, A. (2018). Practice guideline update summary: Mild cognitive impairment: Report of the Guideline Development, Dissemination, and Implementation Subcommittee of the

American Academy of Neurology. *Neurology, 90*(3), 126–135. https://doi.org/10.1212/WNL.0000000000004826

CHAPTER 18: NUTRITION: YOU ARE WHAT YOU EAT

1. https://www.nhlbi.nih.gov/health/educational/lose_wt/BMI/bmicalc.htm
2. Berti, V., Walters, M., Sterling, J., Quinn, C. G., Logue, M., Andrews, R., Matthews, D. C., Osorio, R. S., Pupi, A., Vallabhajosula, S., Isaacson, R. S., de Leon, M. J., & Mosconi, L. (2018). Mediterranean diet and 3-year Alzheimer brain biomarker changes in middle-aged adults. *Neurology, 90*(20), e1789–e1798.
3. Morris, M. C., Tangney, C. C., Wang, Y., Sacks, F. M., Barnes, L. L., Bennett, D. A., & Aggarwal, N. T. (2015). MIND diet slows cognitive decline with aging. *Alzheimer's & Dementia, 11*(9), 1015–1022.
4. Morris, M. C., Tangney, C. C., Wang, Y., Sacks, F. M., Bennett, D. A., & Aggarwal, N. T. (2015). MIND diet associated with reduced incidence of Alzheimer's disease. *Alzheimer's & Dementia, 11*(9), 1007–1014.
5. Keenan, T. D., Agrón, E., Mares, J. A., Clemens, T. E., van Asten, F., Swaroop, A., Chew, E. Y.; AREDS and AREDS2 Research Groups (2020). Adherence to a Mediterranean diet and cognitive function in the Age-Related Eye Disease Studies 1 & 2. *Alzheimer's & Dementia, 16*(6), 831–842.
6. https://www.fda.gov/food/consumers/advice-about-eating-fish
7. Stonehouse, W., Conlon, C. A., Podd, J., Hill, S. R., Minihane, A. M., Haskell, C., & Kennedy, D. (2013). DHA supplementation improved both memory and reaction time in healthy young adults: A randomized controlled trial. *American Journal of Clinical Nutrition, 97*(5), 1134–1143. https://doi.org/10.3945/ajcn.112.053371

8. Dangour, A. D., & Allen, E. (2013). Do omega-3 fats boost brain function in adults? Are we any closer to an answer? *American Journal of Clinical Nutrition, 97*(5), 909–910. https://doi.org/10.3945/ajcn.113.061168

9. Hosseini, M., Poljak, A., Braidy, N., Crawford, J., & Sachdev, P. (2020). Blood fatty acids in Alzheimer's disease and mild cognitive impairment: A meta-analysis and systematic review. *Ageing Research Reviews, 60,* 101043. https://doi.org/10.1016/j.arr.2020.101043.

10. Quinn, J. F., Raman, R., Thomas, R. G.,Yurko-Mauro, K., Nelson, E. B., Van Dyck, C., Galvin, J. E., Emond, J., Jack, C. R. Jr., Weiner, M., Shinto, L., & Aisen, P. S. (2010). Docosahexanoic acid supplementation and cognitive decline in Alzheimer's disease. *JAMA, 304,* 1903–1911.

11. Littlejohns, T. J., Henley, W. E., Lang, I. A., Annweiler, C., Beauchet, O., Chaves, P. H. M., Fried, L., Kestenbaum, B. R., Kuller, L. H., Langa, K. M., Lopez, O. L., Kos, K., Soni, M., & Llewellyn, D. J. (2014). Vitamin D and the risk of dementia and Alzheimer disease. *Neurology, 83,* 920–928.

12. Solomon, P. R., Adams, F., Silver, A., Zimmer, J., & DeVeaux, R. (2002). Ginkgo for memory enhancement: A randomized controlled trial. *JAMA, 288*(7), 835–840. https://doi.org/10.1001/jama.288.7.835

13. Snitz, B. E., O'Meara, E. S., Carlson, M. C., Arnold, A. M., Ives, D. G., Rapp, S. R., Saxton, J., Lopez, O. L., Dunn, L. O., Sink, K. M., DeKosky, S. T., & Ginkgo Evaluation of Memory (GEM) Study Investigators (2009). Ginkgo biloba for preventing cognitive decline in older adults: A randomized trial. *JAMA, 302*(24), 2663–2670. https://doi.org/10.1001/jama.2009.1913

14. Turner, R. S., Thomas, R. G., Craft, S., van Dyck, C. H., Mintzer, J., Reynolds, B. A., Brewer, J. B., Rissman, R. A., Raman, R., Aisen, P. S., & Alzheimer's Disease Cooperative Study (2015). A randomized, double-blind, placebo-controlled trial of resveratrol for Alzheimer disease.

Neurology, *85*(16), 1383–1391. https://doi.org/10.1212/ WNL.0000000000002035

15. https://www.ftc.gov/news-events/press-releases/2017/01/ ftc-new-york-state-charge-marketers-prevagen-making-deceptive

16. Valls-Pedret, C., Sala-Vila, A., Serra-Mir, M., Corella, D., de la Torre, R., Martínez-González, M. Á., Martínez-Lapiscina, E. H., Fitó, M., Pérez-Heras, A., Salas-Salvadó, J., Estruch, R., & Ros, E. (2015). Mediterranean diet and age-related cognitive decline: A randomized clinical trial. *JAMA Internal Medicine, 175*(7), 1094–1103. https://doi.org/ 10.1001/jamainternmed.2015.1668

CHAPTER 19: THIS IS YOUR BRAIN ON ALCOHOL, CANNABIS, AND DRUGS

1. Söderlund, H., Grady, C. L., Easdon, C., & Tulving, E. (2007). Acute effects of alcohol on neural correlates of episodic memory encoding. *NeuroImage, 35*(2), 928–939. https://doi.org/10.1016/j.neuroimage.2006.12.024

2. Solfrizzi, V., D'Introno, A., Colacicco, A. M., Capurso, C., Del Parigi, A., Baldassarre, G., Scapicchio, P., Scafato, E., Amodio, M., Capurso, A., Panza, F., & Italian Longitudinal Study on Aging Working Group (2007). Alcohol consumption, mild cognitive impairment, and progression to dementia. *Neurology, 68*(21), 1790–1799. https://doi.org/ 10.1212/01.wnl.0000262035.87304.89

3. Topiwala, A., & Ebmeier, K. P. (2018). Effects of drinking on late-life brain and cognition. *Evidence-Based Mental Health, 21*(1), 12–15. https://doi.org/10.1136/eb-2017-102820

4. GBD 2016 Alcohol Collaborators. (2018). Alcohol use and burden for 195 countries and territories, 1990-2016: A systematic analysis for the Global Burden of Disease Study

2016. *Lancet, 392*(10152), 1015–1035. https://doi.org/10.1016/S0140-6736(18)31310-2

5. Sewell, R. A., Poling, J., & Sofuoglu, M. (2009). The effect of cannabis compared with alcohol on driving. *American Journal on Addictions, 18*(3), 185–193. https://doi.org/10.1080/10550490902786934

6. https://www.washingtonpost.com/transportation/2020/01/30/proportion-drivers-fatal-crashes-who-tested-positive-thc-doubled-after-marijuanas-legalization-study-finds/

7. Dahlgren, M. K., Sagar, K. A., Smith, R. T., Lambros, A. M., Kuppe, M. K., & Gruber, S. A. (2020). Recreational cannabis use impairs driving performance in the absence of acute intoxication. *Drug and Alcohol Dependence, 208*, 107771. https://doi.org/10.1016/j.drugalcdep.2019.107771

8. Schuster, R. M., Gilman, J., Schoenfeld, D., Evenden, J., Hareli, M., Ulysse, C., Nip, E., Hanly, A., Zhang, H., & Evins, A. E. (2018). One month of cannabis abstinence in adolescents and young adults is associated with improved memory. *Journal of Clinical Psychiatry, 79*(6), 17m11977. https://doi.org/10.4088/JCP.17m11977

9. Pope, H. G., Jr, Gruber, A. J., Hudson, J. I., Huestis, M. A., & Yurgelun-Todd, D. (2001). Neuropsychological performance in long-term cannabis users. *Archives of General Psychiatry, 58*(10), 909–915. https://doi.org/10.1001/archpsyc.58.10.909

10. Platt, B., O'Driscoll, C., Curran, V. H., Rendell, P. G., & Kamboj, S. K. (2019). The effects of licit and illicit recreational drugs on prospective memory: A meta-analytic review. *Psychopharmacology, 236*(4), 1131–1143. https://doi.org/10.1007/s00213-019-05245-9

11. Morgan, C., Freeman, T. P., Hindocha, C., Schafer, G., Gardner, C., & Curran, H. V. (2018). Individual and combined effects of acute delta-9-tetrahydrocannabinol and cannabidiol on psychotomimetic symptoms and memory

function. *Translational Psychiatry, 8*(1), 181. https://doi.org/10.1038/s41398-018-0191-x

12. Curran, T., Devillez, H., York Williams, S. L., & Bidwell, C. L. (2020) Acute effects of naturalistic THC vs. CBD use on recognition memory: A preliminary study. *Journal of Cannabis Research, 2*, 28. https://doi.org/10.1186/s42238-020-00034-0

13. ElSohly, M. A., Mehmedic, Z., Foster, S., Gon, C., Chandra, S., & Church, J. C. (2016). Changes in cannabis potency over the last 2 decades (1995–2014): Analysis of current data in the United States. *Biological Psychiatry, 79*(7), 613–619. https://doi.org/10.1016/j.biopsych.2016.01.004

14. Cuttler, C., LaFrance, E. M., & Stueber, A. (2021). Acute effects of high-potency cannabis flower and cannabis concentrates on everyday life memory and decision making. *Scientific Reports, 11*(1), 13784. https://doi.org/10.1038/s41598-021-93198-5

15. Hotz, J., Fehlmann, B., Papassotiropoulos, A., de Quervain, D. J., & Schicktanz, N. S. (2021). Cannabidiol enhances verbal episodic memory in healthy young participants: A randomized clinical trial. *Journal of Psychiatric Research, 143*, 327–333. https://doi.org/10.1016/j.jpsychires.2021.09.007

16. Gruber, S. A., Sagar, K. A., Dahlgren, M. K., Gonenc, A., Smith, R. T., Lambros, A. M., Cabrera, K. B., & Lukas, S. E. (2018). The grass might be greener: Medical marijuana patients exhibit altered brain activity and improved executive function after 3 months of treatment. *Frontiers in Pharmacology, 8*, 983. https://doi.org/10.3389/fphar.2017.00983

17. Laws, K. R., & Kokkalis, J. (2007). Ecstasy (MDMA) and memory function: A meta-analytic update. *Human Psychopharmacology, 22*(6), 381–388. https://doi.org/10.1002/hup.857

18. Daumann, J., Fischermann, T., Heekeren, K., Henke, K., Thron, A., & Gouzoulis-Mayfrank, E. (2005).

Memory-related hippocampal dysfunction in poly-drug ecstasy (3,4-methylenedioxymethamphetamine) users. *Psychopharmacology, 180*(4), 607–611. https://doi.org/10.1007/s00213-004-2002-8

19. Moon, M., Do, K. S., Park, J., & Kim, D. (2007). Memory impairment in methamphetamine-dependent patients. *International Journal of Neuroscience, 117*(1), 1–9. https://doi.org/10.1080/00207450500535503

20. Gruber, S. A., Tzilos, G. K., Silveri, M. M., Pollack, M., Renshaw, P. F., Kaufman, M. J., & Yurgelun-Todd, D. A. (2006). Methadone maintenance improves cognitive performance after two months of treatment. *Experimental and Clinical Psychopharmacology, 14*(2), 157–164. https://doi.org/10.1037/1064-1297.14.2.157

21. Healy, C. J. (2021). The acute effects of classic psychedelics on memory in humans. *Psychopharmacology, 238*, 639–653. https://doi.org/10.1007/s00213-020-05756-w

CHAPTER 20: SLEEP WELL

1. Cirelli, C., & Tononi, G. (2017). The sleeping brain. *Cerebrum: The Dana Forum on Brain Science, 2017*, cer-07-17.

2. Mander, B. A., Santhanam, S., Saletin, J. M., & Walker, M. P. (2011). Wake deterioration and sleep restoration of human learning. *Current Biology, 21*(5), R183–R184. https://doi.org/10.1016/j.cub.2011.01.019

3. Walker, M. (2017). *Why we sleep.* Scribner.

4. Rudoy, J. D., Voss, J. L., Westerberg, C. E., & Paller, K. A. (2009). Strengthening individual memories by reactivating them during sleep. *Science, 326*(5956), 1079. https://doi.org/10.1126/science.1179013

5. Hu, X., Cheng, L. Y., Chiu, M. H., & Paller, K. A. (2020). Promoting memory consolidation during sleep: A meta-analysis of targeted memory reactivation. *Psychological*

Bulletin, 146(3), 218–244. https://doi.org/10.1037/bul 0000223

6. Sanders, K., Osburn, S., Paller, K. A., & Beeman, M. (2019). Targeted memory reactivation during sleep improves next-day problem solving. *Psychological Science, 30*(11), 1616–1624. https://doi.org/10.1177/0956797619873344

7. Wassing, R., Lakbila-Kamal, O., Ramautar, J. R., Stoffers, D., Schalkwijk, F., & Van Someren, E. (2019). Restless REM sleep impedes overnight amygdala adaptation. *Current Biology, 29*(14), 2351–2358.e4. https://doi.org/10.1016/j.cub.2019.06.034

8. Cartwright, R., Young, M. A., Mercer, P., & Bears, M. (1998). Role of REM sleep and dream variables in the prediction of remission from depression. *Psychiatry Research, 80*(3), 249–255. https://doi.org/10.1016/s0165-1781(98)00071-7

9. Robbins, R., Quan, S. F., Weaver, M. D., Bormes, G., Barger, L. K., & Czeisler, C. A. (2021). Examining sleep deficiency and disturbance and their risk for incident dementia and all-cause mortality in older adults across 5 years in the United States. *Aging, 13*(3), 3254–3268. https://doi.org/10.18632/aging.202591

10. Lim, A. S., Kowgier, M., Yu, L., Buchman, A. S., & Bennett, D. A. (2013). Sleep fragmentation and the risk of incident Alzheimer's disease and cognitive decline in older persons. *Sleep, 36*(7), 1027–1032. https://doi.org/10.5665/sleep.2802

11. Lim, A. S., Yu, L., Kowgier, M., Schneider, J. A., Buchman, A. S., & Bennett, D. A. (2013). Modification of the relationship of the apolipoprotein E ε4 allele to the risk of Alzheimer disease and neurofibrillary tangle density by sleep. *JAMA Neurology, 70*(12), 1544–1551. https://doi.org/10.1001/jamaneurol.2013.4215

12. Patterson, P. D., Ghen, J. D., Antoon, S. F., Martin-Gill, C., Guyette, F. X., Weiss, P. M., Turner, R. L., & Buysse, D. J. (2019). Does evidence support "banking/extending sleep" by shift workers to mitigate fatigue, and/or to improve health,

safety, or performance? A systematic review. *Sleep Health*, 5(4), 359–369. https://doi.org/10.1016/j.sleh.2019.03.001

13. Dewald, J. F., Meijer, A. M., Oort, F. J., Kerkhof, G. A., & Bögels, S. M. (2010). The influence of sleep quality, sleep duration and sleepiness on school performance in children and adolescents: A meta-analytic review. *Sleep Medicine Reviews*, *14*(3), 179–189. https://doi.org/10.1016/j.smrv.2009.10.004

14. Seoane, H. A., Moschetto, L., Orliacq, F., Orliacq, J., Serrano, E., Cazenave, M. I., Vigo, D. E., & Perez-Lloret, S. (2020). Sleep disruption in medicine students and its relationship with impaired academic performance: A systematic review and meta-analysis. *Sleep Medicine Reviews*, *53*, 101333. https://doi.org/10.1016/j.smrv.2020.101333

15. Okano, K., Kaczmarzyk, J. R., Dave, N., Gabrieli, J., & Grossman, J. C. (2019). Sleep quality, duration, and consistency are associated with better academic performance in college students. *NPJ Science of Learning*, *4*, 16. https://doi.org/10.1038/s41539-019-0055-z

16. Huedo-Medina, T. B., Kirsch, I., Middlemass, J., Klonizakis, M., & Siriwardena, A. N. (2012). Effectiveness of non-benzodiazepine hypnotics in treatment of adult insomnia: Meta-analysis of data submitted to the Food and Drug Administration. *BMJ (Clinical Research Ed.)*, *345*, e8343. https://doi.org/10.1136/bmj.e8343

17. https://www.nhlbi.nih.gov/files/docs/public/sleep/healthy_sleep.pdf

CHAPTER 21: ACTIVITIES, ATTITUDE, MUSIC, MINDFULNESS, AND BRAIN TRAINING

1. Matsuzawa, T. (2013). Evolution of the brain and social behavior in chimpanzees. *Current Opinion in Neurobiology*, *23*(3), 443–449. https://doi.org/10.1016/j.conb.2013.01.012

2. Krell-Roesch, J., Syrjanen, J. A., Vassilaki, M., Machulda, M. M., Mielke, M. M., Knopman, D. S., Kremers, W. K., Petersen, R. C., & Geda, Y. E. (2019). Quantity and quality of mental activities and the risk of incident mild cognitive impairment. *Neurology, 93*(6), e548–e558. https://doi.org/10.1212/WNL.0000000000007897

3. James, B. D., Wilson, R. S., Barnes, L. L., & Bennett, D. A. (2011). Late-life social activity and cognitive decline in old age. *Journal of the International Neuropsychological Society, 17*(6), 998–1005. https://doi.org/10.1017/S1355617711000531

4. Wilson, R. S., Boyle, P. A., James, B. D., Leurgans, S. E., Buchman, A. S., & Bennett, D. A. (2014). Negative social interactions and risk of mild cognitive impairment in old age. *Neuropsychology, 29*(4), 561–570. doi:http://dx.doi.org/10.1037/neu0000154

5. Sachs, M. E., Habibi, A., Damasio, A., & Kaplan, J. T. (2020). Dynamic intersubject neural synchronization reflects affective responses to sad music. *NeuroImage, 218*, 116512. https://doi.org/10.1016/j.neuroimage.2019.116512

6. Toiviainen, P., Burunat, I., Brattico, E., Vuust, P., & Alluri, V. (2020). The chronnectome of musical beat. *NeuroImage, 216*, 116191. https://doi.org/10.1016/j.neuroimage.2019.116191

7. Wu, K., Anderson, J., Townsend, J., Frazier, T., Brandt, A., & Karmonik, C. (2019). Characterization of functional brain connectivity towards optimization of music selection for therapy: A fMRI study. *International Journal of Neuroscience, 129*(9), 882–889. https://doi.org/10.1080/00207454.2019.1581189

8. Mehegan, L., & Rainville, G. (2020, June). *Music nourishes and delights: 2020 AARP Music and Brain Health Survey.* https://doi.org/10.26419/res.00387.001

9. Gómez Gallego, M., & Gómez García, J. (2017). Music therapy and Alzheimer's disease: Cognitive, psychological, and

behavioural effects. *Neurologia, 32*(5), 300–308. https://doi. org/10.1016/j.nrl.2015.12.003

10. *Alive Inside: A Story of Music and Memory.* Wikipedia. https://en.wikipedia.org/w/index.php?title=Alive_Inside:_ A_Story_of_Music_and_Memory&oldid=991942258

11. Predovan, D., Julien, A., Esmail, A., & Bherer, L. (2019). Effects of dancing on cognition in healthy older adults: A systematic review. *Journal of Cognitive Enhancement, 3*(2), 161–167. https://doi.org/10.1007/s41465-018-0103-2

12. Echaide, C., Del Río, D., & Pacios, J. (2019). The differential effect of background music on memory for verbal and visuo-spatial information. *Journal of General Psychology, 146*(4), 443–458. https://doi.org/10.1080/00221309.2019.1602023

13. Gallant. S. N. (2016). Mindfulness meditation practice and executive functioning: Breaking down the benefit. *Consciousness and Cognition, 40*, 116–130. https://doi.org/ 10.1016/j.concog.2016.01.005

14. Brown, K. W., Goodman, R. J., Ryan, R. M., & Anālayo, B. (2016). Mindfulness enhances episodic memory perfor-mance: Evidence from a multimethod investigation. *PLoS One, 11*(4), e0153309. doi:10.1371/journal.pone.0153309

15. Isbel, B., Weber, J., Lagopoulos, J., Stefanidis, K., Anderson, H., & Summers, M. J. (2020). Neural changes in early visual processing after 6 months of mindfulness training in older adults. *Scientific Reports, 10*(1), 21163. https://doi.org/ 10.1038/s41598-020-78343-w

16. Levy, B. R., Zonderman, A. B., Slade, M. D., & Ferrucci, L. (2012). Memory shaped by age stereotypes over time. *Journals of Gerontology. Series B, Psychological Sciences and Social Sciences, 67*(4), 432–436. https://doi.org/10.1093/ger onb/gbr120

17. Levy, B. R., & Myers, L. M. (2004). Preventive health behav-iors influenced by self-perceptions of aging. *Preventive Medicine, 39*(3), 625–629. doi:10.1016/j.ypmed.2004.02.029

18. Barber, S. J. (2020). The applied implications of age-based stereotype threat for older adults. *Journal of Applied Research in Memory and Cognition, 9*(3), 274–285, https://doi.org/10.1016/j.jarmac.2020.05.002

19. Steele, C. M., & Aronson, J. (1995). Stereotype threat and the intellectual test performance of African Americans. *Journal of Personality and Social Psychology, 69*, 797–811. doi:10.1037/0022-3514.69.5.797

20. Krell-Roesch, J., Syrjanen, J. A., Vassilaki, M., Machulda, M. M., Mielke, M. M., Knopman, D. S., Kremers, W. K., Petersen, R. C., & Geda, Y. E. (2019). Quantity and quality of mental activities and the risk of incident mild cognitive impairment. *Neurology, 93*(6), e548–e558. https://doi.org/10.1212/WNL.0000000000007897

21. Fritsch, T., Smyth, K. A., Debanne, S. M., Petot, G. J., & Friedland, R. P. (2005). Participation in novelty-seeking leisure activities and Alzheimer's disease. *Journal of Geriatric Psychiatry and Neurology, 18*(3), 134–141. https://doi.org/10.1177/0891988705277537

22. Tranter, L. J., & Koutstaal, W. (2008). Age and flexible thinking: An experimental demonstration of the beneficial effects of increased cognitively stimulating activity on fluid intelligence in healthy older adults. *Aging, Neuropsychology, and Cognition, 15*(2), 184–207. doi:10.1080/13825580701322163

23. Lindstrom, H. A., Fritsch, T., Petot, G., Smyth, K. A., Chen, C. H., Debanne, S. M., Lerner, A. J., & Friedland, R. P. (2005). The relationships between television viewing in midlife and the development of Alzheimer's disease in a case-control study. *Brain and Cognition, 58*(2), 157–165. doi:10.1016/j.bandc.2004.09.020

24. Sharifian, N., & Zahodne, L. B. (2021). Daily associations between social media use and memory failures: The mediating role of negative affect. *Journal of General Psychology, 148*(1), 67–83. doi:10.1080/00221309.2020.1743228

25. Federal Trade Commission. (2015, April 9). *FTC approves final order barring company from making unsubstantiated claims related to products' "brain training" capabilities.* https://www.ftc.gov/news-events/press-releases/2015/04/ftc-appro ves-final-order-barring-company-making-unsubstantiated

26. Federal Trade Commission. (2016, January 5). *Lumosity to pay $2 million to settle FTC deceptive advertising charges for its "Brain Training" program: Company claimed program would sharpen performance in everyday life and protect against cognitive decline.* https://www.ftc.gov/news-events/press-releases/2016/01/lumosity-pay-2-million-settle-ftc-deceptive-advertising-charges

27. West, R. K., Rabin, L. A., Silverman, J. M., Moshier, E., Sano, M., & Beeri, M. S. (2020). Short-term computerized cognitive training does not improve cognition compared to an active control in non-demented adults aged 80 years and above. *International Psychogeriatrics, 32*(1), 65–73. https://doi.org/10.1017/S1041610219000267

28. Lee, H. K., Kent, J. D., Wendel, C., Wolinsky, F. D., Foster, E. D., Merzenich, M. M., & Voss, M. W. (2020). Home-based, adaptive cognitive training for cognitively normal older adults: Initial efficacy trial. *Journals of Gerontology. Series B, Psychological Sciences and Social Sciences, 75*(6), 1144–1154. https://doi.org/10.1093/geronb/gbz073

29. Simons, D. J., Boot, W. R., Charness, N., Gathercole, S. E., Chabris, C. F., Hambrick, D. Z., & Stine-Morrow, E. A. (2016). Do "brain-training" programs work? *Psychological Science in the Public Interest, 17*(3), 103–186. https://doi.org/10.1177/1529100616661983

CHAPTER 22: MEMORY AIDS

1. Brown, P. C., Roediger III, H. L., & McDaniel, M. A. (2014). *Make it stick: The science of successful learning.* Belknap Press, an imprint of Harvard University Press.

2. Lorayne, H. (2010). *Ageless memory: The memory expert's prescription for a razor-sharp mind.* Black Dog & Leventhal.

3. Foer, J. (2011). *Moonwalking with Einstein: The art and science of remembering everything.* Penguin Press.

4. Budson, A. E., & O'Connor, M. K. (2017). *Seven steps to managing your memory: What's normal, what's not, and what to do about it.* Oxford University Press.

5. https://en.wikipedia.org/wiki/Time_management#The_Eisenhower_Method

CHAPTER 25: ADVANCED STRATEGIES AND MNEMONICS

1. Foer, J. (2011). *Moonwalking with Einstein: The art and science of remembering everything.* Penguin Press.

2. https://danielkilov.com/2014/05/05/the-memory-systems-of-mark-twain/

3. https://timeonline.uoregon.edu/twain/pleasures.php

4. https://en.wikipedia.org/wiki/Mnemonic_major_system#History Accessed 4/17/2021

5. Lorayne, H. (2010). *Ageless memory: The memory expert's prescription for a razor-sharp mind.* Black Dog & Leventhal.

6. Brown, P. C., Roediger III, H. L., & McDaniel, M. A. (2014). *Make it stick: The science of successful learning.* Belknap Press, an imprint of Harvard University Press.

7. https://archive.org/details/adcherenniumdera00capluoft/page/218/mode/2up

About the authors

Andrew E. Budson received his bachelor's degree at Haverford College, where he majored in both chemistry and philosophy. After graduating *cum laude* from Harvard Medical School, he was an intern in internal medicine at Brigham and Women's Hospital. He then attended the Harvard-Longwood Neurology Residency Program, for which he was chosen to be chief resident in his senior year. He next pursued a fellowship in behavioral neurology and dementia at Brigham and Women's Hospital, after which he joined the neurology department there. He participated in numerous clinical trials of new drugs to treat Alzheimer's disease in his role as the Associate Medical Director of Clinical Trials for Alzheimer's Disease at Brigham and Women's Hospital. Following his clinical training he spent three years studying memory as a post-doctoral fellow in experimental psychology and cognitive neuroscience at Harvard University under Professor Daniel Schacter. After five years as Assistant Professor of Neurology at Harvard Medical School, he joined the Boston University Alzheimer's Disease Research Center and the Geriatric Research Education Clinical Center (GRECC) at the Bedford Veterans Affairs Hospital. During his five years at the Bedford GRECC he served in several roles, including the Director of Outpatient Services, Associate Clinical Director, and later the overall GRECC Director. In 2010 he moved to the Veterans Affairs Boston Healthcare System, where he is currently the Associate Chief of Staff for Education, Chief of Cognitive & Behavioral Neurology, and Director of the Center for Translational Cognitive

Neuroscience. He is also the overall Associate Director and Leader of Outreach, Recruitment, and Education at the Boston University Alzheimer's Disease Research Center, Professor of Neurology at Boston University School of Medicine, and Lecturer in Neurology at Harvard Medical School. Dr. Budson has had National Institutes of Health and other government research funding since 1998, receiving a National Research Service Award and a Career Development Award (K23) in addition to Research Project (R01) and VA Merit grants. He has given over 750 local, national, and international grand rounds and other academic talks, including at the Institute of Cognitive Neuroscience, Queen Square, London; Berlin, Germany; and Cambridge University, England. He has published 9 books and over 150 papers in peer-reviewed journals, including *The New England Journal of Medicine*, *Brain*, and *Cortex*, and is a reviewer for more than 50 journals. He was awarded the Norman Geschwind Prize in Behavioral Neurology in 2008 and the Research Award in Geriatric Neurology in 2009, both from the American Academy of Neurology. His current research uses the techniques of experimental psychology and cognitive neuroscience to understand memory and memory distortions in patients with Alzheimer's disease and other neurological disorders. In his Memory Disorders Clinic at the Veterans Affairs Boston Healthcare System he treats patients while teaching medical students, residents, and fellows. He also sees patients at the Boston Center for Memory in Newton, Massachusetts. When not working or writing, he enjoys spending time with his family, traveling, running, skiing, kayaking, biking, and practicing yoga.

Elizabeth A. Kensinger is currently Professor and Chairperson of the Department of Psychology and Neuroscience at Boston College, where she has directed the Cognitive and Affective Neuroscience laboratory since 2006. She graduated *summa cum laude* from Harvard University, with a joint degree in psychology and biology, and she completed a Ph.D. in neuroscience at the Massachusetts Institute of Technology, supported by a Howard Hughes Medical Institute Predoctoral Fellowship. After post-doctoral training at Harvard University and the Massachusetts General Hospital, supported by fellowships from the Massachusetts Biomedical Research Corporation and the National Institute of Mental Health, she secured her faculty appointment at Boston College. There, she teaches courses on human memory and affective neuroscience, and engages students in research practice. Over the years she has mentored dozens of post-doctoral fellows and graduate students, and over 100 undergraduate students. Most of her laboratory members have gone on to careers in academia, but she can tout that her undergraduate research assistants have leveraged their training for use in careers literally ranging from A (advertising) to Z (zoology). Dr. Kensinger has published over 200 research articles and has served as Associate Editor of *Emotion* and *Cognition and Emotion*, and as a founding Associate Editor of *Affective Science*. She has received awards from the Cognitive Neuroscience Society, the Association for Psychological Science, and the American Psychological Association, and she had the honor of serving as Chair of the Program Committee for the former two societies. Her research is funded by the National Science Foundation and the National Institutes of Health, and her laboratory also has recently been supported by funding from the McKnight Endowment Fund for Neuroscience, the Retirement Research Foundation, and the American Federation for Aging Research. Her laboratory also has benefited from a gift by members of the Boston College Class of 1991 to support research on learning and memory conducted to improve the educational experience for students with memory challenges. Her research combines multiple methods (functional magnetic resonance imaging, event-related potentials, polysomnography, psychophysiology, eye-tracking) to answer questions such as: Why do we remember some moments from our past, such as those imbued with emotion, better than others? Why is sleep so important for memory? How does memory change as adults get older, and what can we do to minimize the negative impact of those changes? When not in the laboratory or classroom, she is most likely to be found baking and decorating cakes or spending time outdoors with her husband and daughter. They especially enjoy spending time in the mountains of New England, where their daughter is sometimes challenged to keep pace on hikes up the mountains, and Elizabeth is always challenged to catch up with their daughter while skiing down them.

Index